Science Education
and
Ethical Values

Science Education and Ethical Values

Introducing Ethics and Religion into the Science Classroom and Laboratory

Edited by
Bert Musschenga and David Gosling

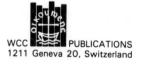

WCC PUBLICATIONS
1211 Geneva 20, Switzerland

GEORGETOWN UNIVERSITY PRESS
Washington, D.C., 20057, USA

Published for the WCC Sub-unit on Church and Society and the
Free University of Amsterdam by WCC Publications, Geneva,
in collaboration with Georgetown University Press,
Washington, DC 20057, USA
ISBN 2-8254-0811-5 (WCC)
ISBN 0-87840-420-1 (GUP)

Library of Congress Cataloging in Publication Data
Main entry under title:

Science education and ethical values.

   Includes proceedings of a workshop organized by the World Council of Churches
and the Free University of Amsterdam, held June 20-24, 1983 at the University.
   1. Science—Study and teaching—Moral and ethical aspects—Congresses.
I. Musschenga, Bert. II. Gosling, David L., 1939-   . III. World Council of
Churches. IV. Vrije Universiteit te Amsterdam.
Q181.A1S34 1985   174'.95'071   84-28599
ISBN 0-87840-420-1

Cover design: Michael M. Dominguez
© 1985 World Council of Churches, 150, route de Ferney
1211 Geneva 20, Switzerland

Typeset by Thomson Press (India) Ltd., New Delhi
Printed in Switzerland

CONTENTS

Introduction vi

Dominant Scientific Methodological Views: Alternatives and Their
Implications *David Edge* 1

Religion, Values and Science Education *Ian G. Barbour* 10

Values, Responsibilities and Commitments in the Teaching of Science
Charles Birch 20

Moral Development and Education *Gerhard Portele* 31

Reasoning in Science and Ethics *Gerrit Manenschijn* 37

Collective Social Decision-Making: Implications for Teaching Science
Glen S. Aikenhead 55

Ethics in the Classroom: Goals and Experiences *Harrie Eijkelhof* . 68

Implementing Educational Innovations *Alfred K.F. Schermer* . . . 79

Science Education and Society
 Summary of the Discussion *Howard Davis* 90
 Report 93

Science Education in Universities
 Summary of the Discussion *Henk Verhoog* 98
 Report 101

Science Education in Secondary Schools and Teacher Training
Institutes: Integrated Report 107

List of Participants 112

INTRODUCTION

From 20 to 24 June 1983, forty delegates assembled at the student centre of the Free University of Amsterdam in the Netherlands to discuss means of integrating moral and ethical concerns into science education. The majority were from Western Europe (Sweden, Finland, Denmark, Great Britain, Federal Republic of Germany, the Netherlands, Italy and Spain), though other countries such as India, Kenya, the USA, Indonesia and Australia, were also represented.

The workshop was the first in what is hoped to be a series on science education and ethics organized by the World Council of Churches jointly with the Free University of Amsterdam in collaboration with different partners from various parts of the world. The Free University of Amsterdam is a Protestant Christian higher educational institution committed to educational issues many of which are on the agenda of the ecumenical movement. The theme "Science Education and Ethics" was a logical follow-up of the WCC 1979 conference on "Faith, Science and the Future" held at the Massachusetts Institute of Technology and the Free University's 1980 celebration of its first centennial based on the theme "Concern about Science". During the latter conference the then rector magnificus, Dr H. Verheul, discussed with representatives of the WCC and members of his own university the possibility of a joint workshop on science education and ethics. These discussions ultimately gave birth to the workshop the proceedings of which constitute much of the subject matter of this book. Differences in cultural background, in socio-political context and in educational systems are important when one considers what has to be done to introduce ethical issues into science education. Since the Free University is in Western Europe, it was decided to hold the first regional workshop there.

The fact that the workshop was to concentrate on the integration of ethics with science education, and not in the first place on ethical reflection itself, had implications for its structure, the subjects to be discussed and the speakers and participants to be invited. The speakers were experts either on more theoretical questions such as moral reasoning, collective decision-making, the methodology of science, science and religion and moral development, or more practical questions such as development and the testing of new teaching materials and curriculum developments. Those invited as participants had to be involved in science education, or else were experts in a discipline related to science education (e.g. ethics, psychology, philosophy of science). The intention was to have as participants not only science educators working at universities, but also teacher trainers and persons working at institutes which develop teaching materials and curricula for secondary schools. It is widely recognized that the standard picture of science is fixed in the minds of pupils at the secondary school level. Those present at the workshop were a mix of people representing many disciplines. The preparatory committee did not succeed in finding participant-observers from Eastern Europe; there were only three people from the third world and the number of women was relatively small.

The atmosphere throughout the workshop was stimulating, and the discussions were thoughtful and productive. The participants felt that concentration on problems and preconditions for the integration of ethical discussions in science education made the workshop particularly useful, and ultimately concluded that the improvement of science education is the responsibility of both educational institutions and the churches.

The workshop became especially interesting as attempts were made to translate changes in understandings on matters related to science and education into consequences for the form and content of science education.

Firstly, the change in the image of science from one in which science is considered to be value-free or value-neutral to one in which it is viewed as value-laden: how contextual (social, political) values influence different stages of scientific research (choice of the subject of research; the building of hypotheses, etc.). Thus it is important for pupils to get a realistic picture of science.

Secondly, the growing awareness that the impact of science and technology on society and individuals is not necessarily beneficial, and the implications of this for the picture of science that is usually presented to pupils and students.

Thirdly, the discovery of many scientists and science students that science cannot answer questions about the meaning of existence in general and of their own lives in particular. Related to this is the realization that the view that only scientific ways of knowing lead to valid knowledge about reality effectively blocks the entrance to other fields of knowledge. Students must learn and experience for themselves that there are many forms of knowledge of which scientific knowledge is only one.

Fourthly, the emphasis of modern education on the development of a broad range of capacities of pupils rather than on the learning of specific skills as such. An important corollary is that science education must focus more on teaching how to use scientific knowledge and skills in personal and social life.

Fifthly, while for along time science has been seen as rational and objective, and ethics as non-rational, relativistic and subjective, we now increasingly regard science as less objective and rational, and ethics more so. This new way of looking at the nature of ethical knowledge has consequences for the manner in which we discuss ethical and political problems related to science and technology in science education. It is not sufficient for pupils and students to learn to express their views, they must also learn that one has to justify them and how to do so.

Sixthly, a further important facet of science education is that many if not most ethical and social problems necessitate collective decisions. Therefore moral education cannot stop at the level of individual judgments, but must also direct itself to the question of how groups or society as a whole can decide on problems about which people fundamentally disagree.

David Edge set out three models of science education which reflect different views of the nature and methods of science: the so-called "product", "inquiry" and "relevance" models. The "product" model aims to impart an unproblematic body of knowledge about the natural world; the "inquiry model" aims to satisfy curiosity about the way the world is; the "relevance model" aims to acquire knowledge for the sake of collective liberation and personal development. These views on the aims of science education correspond with views on the nature of the teacher/student relation. The "product model" is the dominant one; the other two are the "alternatives". According to Edge it is an open question whether the alternatives should be integrated into science education, and whether they can be. He drew attention to the fact that a preference for one of the models does not only depend on epistemological views, but also on moral ideas and on views on education in general. The second model is desirable because "thinking scientifically" is often held to be a moral virtue. The third model presupposes the view that the aim of education is individual development and emancipation. Science education should also contribute to that aim. Application of that model has political implications also because it requires the restructuring of the relations of power and authority, both within educational institutions and in society at large. He himself preferred mixing the three models, but he doubts whether such a compromise is possible when one takes into account the fact that the dominant model is connected with power structures and vested interests.

In the many presentations and discussions one could often notice the idea that the dominant (i.e. empiricist and positivist) view on the nature and methods of science—its claims to lead to objective knowledge—does not give a realistic picture of science. Science is always linked to interests and is invariably influenced by contextual values. If those values are not made explicit then they exert a hidden influence. Both Ian Barbour and Charles Birch discussed the materialistic impact that the study of science often seems to have on the outlook of students. As Barbour stated, this may partly be the result of a preoccupation with science to the exclusion of other areas of interest and experience. It may also be a product of the attempt to rely exclusively on the methods of science. It is the responsibility of science teachers to convey to students some sense of the limitations of the methods of science and some humility concerning the tentative and selective character of scientific theories. According to Birch "conventional valid science" tries to understand the world by reducing it to its basic physical properties such as atoms or their parts and then tries to build up a world from these "building blocks"—the "substance" model, as he called it.

Science based on the "substance" model is geared to technological application. Birch proposed an alternative, viz. the ecological model. The basic principle of this model is that we understand that which is not ourselves by analogy with what we know ourselves to be. Not only humans, but all entities have subjective experiences and internal relations. Science can never say the final word about entities, because science is studying objects, and entities are subjects. A science education based on that insight can never present scientific knowledge as certain and value-free. The ecological model takes away the blockage that makes a dialogue between science and religion so difficult.

Not only changes in the image of science but also changed ideas on the goals of science education have consequences for the teaching of science. It was generally agreed that transmission of science should be only one of the goals of science education; the importance of that goal depends on the level of the educational system. The goals of science education are influenced by developments in the general aims of education. If moral education is seen as a legitimate part of education, then we must ask how science education can make a contribution.

Gerhard Portele considers that the existing contribution of science education to moral education is not very positive. The results of his research point to a negative correlation between the level of standardization of a scientific discipline and the moral stage (as defined in Kohlberg's theory of the stages of moral development) of the scientists. Standardization is defined as the degree to which the behaviour of researchers and teachers in a discipline can be predicted by the material and the knowledge of the material they deal with. Natural sciences are more standardized than social sciences, and natural scientists show a relatively low stage of moral development.

It is not enough to make the picture of science underlying science education more realistic and to show that science is influenced by society and has an impact on all kinds of social issues. The problem remains how to deal with those issues in science education and how one should discuss the role of science either in causing or in solving them. How should an ethical discussion on social issues be structured in science education? What is the role of the teacher in that kind of discussion? As Gerrit Manenschijn argued, a standard picture of science does not merely impede the integration of ethical discussions in science education. Also a standard picture of ethics exists which describes ethics as subjective, non-rational and relativistic. Within that view of ethics, rational discussions on the ethical aspects of social issues are impossible.

Manenschijn contends that a rational discussion of ethical problems is possible: there are more parallels between moral reasoning and scientific reasoning than the popular views hold. For example, both forms of reasoning presuppose conceptions of the natural world that need to be realistic and workable. Those conceptions must be open for public criticism, which is a methodological as well as a moral requirement. Both forms of reasoning aim at consensus. Choosing subjects of scientific research is a social choice requiring a (moral) concept of a good and just society and (moral) standards of fair decision procedures. The main difference between moral and scientific reasoning is that in moral reasoning the possibility of fundamental disagreement exists, and this cannot be solved by rational argumentation. Such disagreements can refer to differences in the ordering of the basic principles one adheres to. Basic principles are selected, and their choice can only be justified from the perspective of the way of life one wants to live. A way of life is a matter of individual preference; ultimately, basic moral principles rest on preferences for a certain way of life that need not be exclusively rational.

Scientists often must make ethical decisions. It is therefore important for them to know something about moral reasoning. In many social issues science plays an important role, sometimes as the cause of a problem, in other cases in solving a problem. Social issues have to do with the interests of groups of people. This necessarily implies that decisions taken in relation to them must be collective. Problems within the private sphere of life usually require only individual decisions. Different moral views on those problems can exist side by side without conflict. In collective choices on social issues differences in moral opinions necessitate compromises. Most science students will never become scientists, though they will meet science in relation to the social problems for which they bear responsibility as citizens. Therefore it is important that they learn the fundamental tenets of collective decision-making, and this cannot be done only via science education though it can at least teach them how the basic principles of collective decision-making can be applied to problems associated with science and technology.

Collective decision-making on social issues was the subject of Glen Aikenhead's presentation. He underlined the importance of insights into the characteristics and limitations of science and technology. Not only science, but several other knowledge systems (e.g. law, politics, religion, ethics) are potential contributors to collective decision-making. Each social domain has its own tradition and procedures for decision-making. For students and pupils it is fundamental to identify which domain and/or agency has the authority to make an ultimate decision on a specific issue. They should also learn to list plausible alternative solutions, to predict short-term and long-term con-sequences of the several alternatives and to evaluate them against the background of the different values relevant to an issue.

If schools are to be responsible for moral education how should they proceed and what must be their aims? Which skills, competences and attitudes must be developed in order to achieve those aims? Harrie Eijkelhof discussed those questions in the first part of his presentation. The next question was of course how those aims can be realized and what should be the contribution of science education. When one wants to integrate ethics into science education, what will be the consequences for students, teachers, teacher trainers, the curriculum, etc.? Several institutes in countries in Europe and in the USA have developed projects in which ethical aspects are integrated. Eijkelhof summarized his experiences with projects of the Dutch institute, PLON (Project Curriculum Development Physics).

The introduction of social issues often meets resistance not only from schools boards and teachers, but also from students. Because many social issues are quite controversial from a political point of view school board and other official bodies often fear political indoctrination. They are afraid that teachers will preach their own political convictions, and will not give impartial and objective information. In their view there are only two alternatives: objective information and indoctrination. They do not realize the importance of a degree of training in moral reasoning and collective decision-making geared to the development of the students' *own* standpoints. Teachers often resist discussion of social issues because they themselves can play no role other than that of the expert. Students often regard such discussions as marginal to "real" science education.

Many innovative ideas were discussed. But, as Alfred Schermer stated, new ideas are only the first step. The adoption and implementation of such ideas are the more difficult steps. Adoption is the decision to accept a certain idea, innovation or curriculum and to put it into practice. Implementation is the way in which innovations etc. are put into practice. Changes in a curriculum have several dimensions: subject matter or material, organizational structure, role/behaviour, knowledge and understanding and value internalization. Innovation, therefore, is a very complex process. Schermer proceeded to review the various factors that influence adoption and implementation, such as the clarity of innovative proposals, their complexity in the five dimensions of change, the presence of in-service training for teachers, the availability of new teaching materials and the degree of participation of the teachers in the development of new curricula.

The presentations of the various speakers gave an important stimulus to discussions in the working groups. There were many understandable parallels between the discussions of the teacher training group and those of the class-room teaching group—after all, one cannot consider changes in the training of teachers without a clear view of science education in secondary schools. And *vice versa*, the changes in the aims, the methodology and the content of science education on the secondary level have implications for the training of teachers. The discussions in these two groups focused more directly on the pedagogical and educational aspects of the integration of ethics in science education than in the other two groups. It is a well known fact that teachers at secondary schools and teacher trainers pay more attention to didactic problems than university teachers. Perhaps the didactic problems are more urgent at those levels, but university teachers can learn from the experiences of teachers trainers and science teachers at secondary schools. On the other hand science teachers and teacher trainers must learn from critical thinking in universities about science and its limitations. In one of its recommendations the university group mentions the theological faculties, underlining their responsibility to pay attention to the relation between faith and science and ethical issues in relation to science and technology. It is crucially important for theologians to have some idea of the characteristics and the limitations of the natural sciences and learn how to relate faith (theology) and science on both epistemological and ethical levels.

Many misunderstandings of science and the relation between science and religion exist among the public. As is reported by the working group on the issues of science education related to the general public, there is a need for institutes equipped to promote communication between scientists, technologists and the general public. The formation of such multidisciplinary institutes is the responsibility of universities and churches.

We hope that by means of this book the ideas and experiences of the workshop will be communicated to a large group, especially those involved in science education. As stated earlier this workshop was a Western European undertaking. It is the intention of the World Council of Churches and the Free University to make possible the organization of similar workshops in other parts of the world.

Acknowledgments

The organizing committee of the workshop was chaired initially by Dr H Verheul, professor of physics, and later by Dr Piet Born, lecturer in physics. The secretary was Dr A.W. Musschenga, Head of the Interdisciplinary Centre for the Study of Science, Society and Religion (Bezinningscentrum). Other committee members were Dr E. Boeker, professor of physics, Dr P.P. Kirschenmann, professor in the philosophy of science, the Rev. S. de Lange, student chaplain, Dr P. Licht, lecturer in the teacher training department of the Faculty of Physics, Dr A.K.F. Schermer, lecturer in the teacher training department of the Faculty of Biology, Dr I. Simmers, professor of geology, Mr G. Rot, and Dr H. van der Velden—all of the Free University of Amsterdam.

Among these special credit must be given to Piet Born and Bert Musschenga, and to Dr Paul Abrecht, formerly Director of Church and Society of the World Council of Churches.

DOMINANT SCIENTIFIC METHODOLOGICAL VIEWS: ALTERNATIVES AND THEIR IMPLICATIONS

DAVID EDGE

Although I teach science students, I do not teach them science; and my excursions into ethical discussion are not based on any professional training in such matters. My main interest is in the incorporation into science education of what has become known as "Science, Technology and Society (or STS) Studies". I therefore approach my topic from this perspective.

Before getting to the main substance of what I want to say, two preliminary, and fairly lengthy, remarks are necessary.

Fact and value

The first concerns the difficulty of separating matters of "fact" and of "value". My own professional concerns lie in the sociology of scientific knowledge, and (in teaching) contemporary social issues related to science and technology. To me, the "ethics" in all this is *endemic*: it is an intimate *part* of the constitution of science itself. After all, scientific knowledge arises from a sequence of (essentially social) choices, and therefore constantly reflects social values, even if those values are often "coded" and disguised. No one should be surprised that ethical issues are always present within the discourse of social debate and decision-making. As David Pearce[1] rightly says: "The nuclear debate is about values." But, of course, that debate is *also* about technical details *and* about definitions of "safety" *and* about economics *and* about politics (and a lot else besides) *all at the same time*. No clear separation of "value" questions, which can be discussed quasi-independently, is possible. Indeed, one of the major (ethical?) criticisms of nuclear decisions is that they do tend to be made in this "differentiated", piecemeal way. Bureaucrats and technical experts tend to define the choices, and "set the agenda", so as to encourage this form of "rationality". Recently, advocates of nuclear power have used quantitative "risk assessment" techniques to justify their claim that nuclear power is "acceptably safe". This can be seen as a manipulation of the definition of "rationality": those who do not accept the apparent implication

---

1. "The Nuclear Debate is About Values", *Nature*, Vol. 274, 20 July 1978, p. 200.

of the figures are dubbed "irrational", and their views can be discounted. (Pearce fears that such tactics may extrude crucial values from expression in the public debate.) However, if this tactic *is* a "manipulation", then its analysis and exposure require *both* "technical" *and* "ethical" criticism. The full repertoire of discourses must be simultaneously developed, if the debate is to do justice to the issue. To use W.W. Lowrance's example,[2] we should be able to understand why it may be "rational" *both* to *accept* the (very high) risks of snowmobiles *and* to *reject* the (apparently very much lower) risks of nuclear power.

My point is directly relevant to our theme, for it is often assumed that "ethics" can be introduced into science education by *separate* instruction and discussion. As it happens, I myself *do* teach science students some separate "ethical packets". Topics such as attempts to derive a universal ethic from scientific practice, evolutionary (and ecological) ethics, obligations to future generations, and animal rights, can all be "taught" *in vacuo*, and students happily discuss the ethical issues raised by (for instance) *in vitro* fertilization and animal experimentation. But the challenge to science education is more radical than this. Essentially, the challenge is to "teach science as it is" when "as it is" involves viewing "scientific facts" as *value-laden*. (I will return to this view of science later.) For my overall aim is to help science students to appreciate the ethical dilemmas and values *implicit in the activity*, and in the results and situations to which scientific research gives rise. We try to "tease out" these values—and, of course, expose and discuss the students' own values. Science education then becomes the *context* of ethical education. Clearly, conventional science education does not have this character.

Paradigms

For my second preliminary remark, I must refer to the brief given me by the workshop organizers. I was asked to respond to these questions:

> What is the prevailing paradigm of scientific research? What is the criticism? Teaching of sciences both at university and high-school level takes the current paradigm for granted. Are there alternatives? How could other paradigms be integrated properly in teaching?

Now, it seems to me that this kind of language, which is very widespread, contains a serious misunderstanding of Thomas Kuhn's notion of "paradigm". Paradigms are embedded in *technical practice*. They are *exemplary achievements*—specific, concrete *problem solutions*, which have gained universal acceptance throughout their particular scientific fields as exemplifying valid procedures, and as models of valid procedures for pedagogic use. Paradigms constitute the framework for puzzle-solving "normal science".

---

2. *Of Acceptable Risk: Science and the Determination of Safety*, William Kaufmann, Inc., 1976.

(The Crick/Watson DNA paper is often cited as a "paradigm paradigm".) Each established science has "paradigms", which concretize the accepted knowledge of, and what it is to gain knowledge of, those particular features of the world with which that science is concerned. So we may talk of "paradigms of physics", "paradigms of molecular biology", and so on. The "alternatives" to *them* would be "unaccepted science" (or "deviant science"). I cannot believe that anyone seriously thinks that science education should be based on practices and exemplars that scientists do not accept as legitimate.

Of course, each paradigmatic exemplar may *imply* matters of methodology, epistemology, and the like—but it is not a paradigm *of* those things. A "paradigm *of scientific research*" would be embedded in the technical practice of a discipline whose job it is to observe, analyze and investigate *scientific research*, as its object of study—that is, presumably, the philosophy, history, sociology and psychology of science. But these are (notoriously) "immature" sciences, characterized by a wide variety of beliefs and practices, with no unifying consensus, and little activity analogous to Kuhnian "normal science". Occasional pockets of coherence may emerge (such as in recent work in the sociology of scientific knowledge). But what we have is a range of candidate philosophies and conceptualizations of science—a veritable bricoleur's box of resources, a rich "do-it-yourself" identikit. Some models are rationalist, some inductivist or empiricist, some idealist, some Marxist, some hypothetico-deductive (Popper), some paradigm-based (Kuhn), and some anarchistic (Feyerabend). European philosophers of science offer variations on these, often influenced by social anthropology. Recently, there has been something of a revival in realist philosophies of science. Relevant empirical studies have also entered the debate. History provides an abundance of exemplary tales. Then, by way of Wittgenstein, Hesse, and "theory-laden facts", we now have a flourishing sociology of scientific knowledge. American ("Mertonian") sociology of science offers us analysis of scientists' norms and values, and of differentiation, reward and status in the scientific community; and psychologists have chipped in with their own observations of scientists' behaviour. The result is that the "philosophical" debate is enriched by empirically-based criticism of the simpler notions of empiricism and realism.

There is, then, no one "paradigm of scientific research": instead, we have abundant resources for *post hoc* rationalization! But is there one "dominant view", implicit in the majority of science education? My own nomination would be a lazy empiricism/realism. Certainly, there is a set of powerful myths, still current and active, about the objectivity and value-neutrality of scientific findings, and about (for instance) prediction, testing and falsification in scientific research. "Crucial experiments" are held to be both possible and decisive; classification and "discovery" to be unproblematic in character and realist in essence. All these (and many more) implicit beliefs *suffuse* science education, and constitute its "tacit culture". And all can now be empirically challenged.

We can, therefore (and shortly will), discuss the various *implicit emphases* of models underlying approaches in science education, and indicate briefly the authorities cited in justification of these emphases.

I should add that I take "alternatives" to mean, *not* "imaginative alternatives" (the "wouldn't it be nice if" science were recast like this or that, which currently it isn't), but *alternative descriptions and characterizations* of science *as it is currently practised*—that is to say, alternative "theories" of scientists' research behaviour. And it seems to me a moot point as to whether science teaching either *should* or *could* be recast so as to be "integrated properly" with these alternative conceptions of science "as it really is". As Stephen Brush[3] pointedly asks: "Should the History of Science be Rated X?" The workshop should not too quickly assume that the answer to that question as negative!

Three models

Following the analysis of Judith and Tony Hargreaves,[4] which I have found very helpful and stimulating, I would like to outline three crude "models" of science education, and discuss some of their implications.

THE "PRODUCT" MODEL

There is no evidence that any significant amount of science education at tertiary level differs in essence from Kuhn's[5] characterization (see also Barnes[6]). Students are induced into "normal science" by a gradual introduction to exemplary problem solutions and techniques. It is normally assumed that, to every question, there is "one correct answer". The process is, in Basil Bernstein's terms,[7] devised on a "collection code" with "strong classification and framing": there is a segmented syllabus, and strong boundaries between elements. Teacher/student relationships are hierarchical, and the intention is to maximize the flow of (essentially unproblematic) "facts" and information (i.e. the "products" of science) *from* teacher *to* student. This mode of science education is usually allied to a realist and empiricist-inductivist view of science methodology: the view is commonly implicit, and the realism usually "naive" rather than "critical". Recent criticisms of this model of science (in particular,

---

3. "Should the History of Science be Rated X?", *Science*, Vol. 183, 22 March 1974, pp. 1164–72.
4. "Some Models of School Science in British Curriculum Projects, and Their Implications for STS Teaching at the Secondary Level", *Social Studies of Science*, Vol. 13, No. 4, November 1983.
5. T.S. Kuhn, *The Structure of Scientific Revolutions*, University of Chicago Press, 1962, 2nd ed. 1970.
6. B. Barnes, *T.S. Kuhn and Social Science*, Macmillan, 1982, pp. 16–40.
7. "On the Classification and Framing of Education Knowledge", *Class: Codes and Control*, Routledge & Kegan Paul, 1971, pp. 202–230.

the introduction of elements of pluralism and relativism) seem not to have penetrated or influenced tertiary practice.

In a science education conducted on these principles, students *may* engage in STS studies and ethical reflection, but these aspects are merely studied and examined as further, separate elements in a "collection code" syllabus: the strong boundaries remain. Any move towards an "integrated code" would alter the power relationships between teachers and students, and hence be seen as threatening. (Indeed, the problem of *power and authority* within the educational system—and its relationship to curriculum content, disciplinary identities, ideological justifications and "myths" of science—seems to me to be central to any analysis of the possibilities of, and restrictions on, innovation in science education.) STS or ethical components in such an education have to be justified in strictly utilitarian terms: will they "help" (for example) in the management of R&D, or in the resolution of ethical dilemmas (perhaps to ease public relations?), or just in "doing research better". Any suggestion that these components might be *reflexive*, and assist students to criticize the process in which they are engaged (and the values of this utilitarianism), is firmly extruded.

This is, of course, the familiar "mechanistic" model of science education, purveying "alienated knowledge", that can itself be criticized on ethical grounds. I gather that it was the object of fierce criticism from science students and recent graduates at the 1979 WCC conference at MIT—and that this workshop is a response to just that criticism! Anyone who teaches science students in more "reflexive" contexts knows how this model forms their expectations and reactions. But Kuhn did *not* see his characterization as a *criticism* of the process—quite the contrary. Kuhn saw it (in my view, quite legitimately) as an efficient way to "concentrate attention", as it were—to produce "focused researchers", well equipped to "articulate the paradigm" and hence advance "normal science". And, somewhat paradoxically, this process *hastens* creative innovations, since it maximizes the chance that anomalies will not only arise, but provoke radical reconceptualizations (for a discussion of this point, see Barnes[8]). Whatever one's romantic sympathies may lead one to think, "creativity" is *not* necessarily enhanced by "teaching all the alternatives".

One key question is: could it be otherwise? Are there *any* practical "alternatives" to this kind of training? Surely it must always remain a central feature of science education? Is it *possible* to "integrate" criticisms of the realist/empiricist views into the training of scientists? At the very least, any suggested reforms must pay attention, not only to the possible benefits of change, but also to the *harm* that could be done, through disturbing this proven system. And how can such criticisms be "taught" to the lay public? How *can*

8. *Op. cit.*, pp. 19–20.

we "remove the inappropriate myths"? This leads us naturally to the second model.

THE "INQUIRY" MODEL

Many recent experiments in secondary (and, to some extent, tertiary) science education have stressed the *discovery process*, and hence modified the simpler views summarized above. Emphasis then shifts from the idea that "science" consists of a "body of knowledge" (a "product") to be "transmitted" from teacher to student: rather, it is seen as a potentially generalizable *mode of inquiry*, a process of *rational exploration*. The idea that science is endemically *pluralistic*, and its truth claims are only *relative*, can (at least to some extent) be accommodated in this view. Syllabuses based on these principles lessen the hierarchical division between teachers and students. They are often specifically justified by appeal to the work of Karl Popper, whose hypothetico-deductive view of science methodology provides a rationale for the pedagogy, and its pluralism. (Kuhn and his precursor, Michael Polanyi, are also often cited in support, since both these authors stress the importance of "tacit" elements in the practice of science.) Science education conducted on these lines can move towards an "integrated code": science, STS and ethics share (to at least some extent) a common liberal/humanitarian perspective.

At the secondary level, this approach is usually seen as the most promising for teaching "science for non-scientists"—that is, for "the rest". I sense some impatience with these "discovery methods" in training *future scientists*, for they can often appear "inefficient". And, however "open" the methods may seem, and however much initiative is accorded the student, it is still assumed that there is "one correct answer" at every point: students have got "to end up in the right place"! What would a teacher do with a student who used these discovery methods to devise a genuine "alternative science"? Teachers still firmly control the process, and its assessment. For this reason, there is little scope for reflexivity in STS studies.

THE "RELEVANCE" MODEL

A third generative notion, often held by science teachers (especially at secondary level), stresses the relevance of science to individual development and community needs. Here, "science" encompasses both results and methods. This notion is student-centred: the "science" that is "learned" develops outwards from the student's individual interests and idiosyncracies, and is influenced by many contingent factors. Ideally, the status of the student in teacher/student interaction is at least on a par with the teacher. Teachers can no longer control the process via assessment, since whether "success" is achieved is for individuals and communities to decide. Again, Kuhn and

9. *Against Method: Outline of an Anarchistic Theory of Knowledge*, Humanities Press and New Left Books, 1975.

Polanyi are cited in support: but some see in the work of Paul Feyerabend[9] the strongest justification for this approach. "Science" is seen as (in Feyerabend's terms) "anarchistic", a selective product of many contingencies, and not as a solid and reliable "corpus of knowledge" to be transmitted. Where teachers hold this view of science and its methodology, STS studies and ethical issues can be treated in a fully "integrated" way, as a *constitutive* part of the scientific process. The increase in "self-awareness" and "critical consciousness" which are basic aims in this approach can lead to an emphasis on the more radical, political, and "reflexive" aspects of STS. However, to my knowledge, this notion has not yet been embodied satisfactorily and coherently in any syllabus innovations—although, several years ago, an experimental MIT physics degree was launched on these lines, and the idea obviously underlies the Dutch "science shop" and "transformation of science" initiatives. Individual school-teachers successfully adopt this approach with "drop-outs" and "also-rans". But whether it can successfully replace and transform the "product" model as the *dominant* method in science education *as a whole* is highly doubtful.

Table I summarizes many of these points (see following page).

It is worth noting that the second and third of these models are often justified, not on epistemological, but on *moral* grounds: the second ("inquiry") because "thinking scientifically" is often held to be a moral virtue; the third ("relevance") because it aims to use science for individual development and liberation. And the third is also (and usually) justified on *political* grounds. The latter point is significant because it emphasizes that the fundamental problem in instituting reforms of science education lies not in devising new syllabuses and pedagogical methods, but in *restructuring relations of power and authority*—and not only within educational institutions, but in society at large, for the former is a reflection of the latter. The content and myths of science themselves play a role in consolidating and justifying the power relations in society. This is both the central insight of STS, and the central reason why that insight is so difficult to disseminate!

Science as social convention

In recent years, sociologists and historians of science have developed, through empirical studies in the sociology of scientific knowledge, a still more radical notion of the nature of science and its methods (for an introduction and references, see Mulkay[10] and Barnes and Edge[11]). Its epistemology is Feyerabendian: its stance is close to ethnomethodology. Scientific facts, claims, theories, and the like, are held to be the outcomes of *social negotiations*, in which no "observation of nature" can be unproblematically assumed to have a preferred or decisive role. "Scientific truth" is *actively constructed*;

10. M. Mulkay, *Science and the Sociology of Knowledge*, George Allen & Unwin, 1979.
11. B. Barnes & D. Edge, *Science in Context: Readings in the Sociology of Science*, Open University Press and MIT Press, 1982.

TABLE I: MODELS OF THE SCIENCE CURRICULUM, AND ASSOCIATED STS STUDIES

Model	Aims	Perceptions of science	Teacher/student relationship	Type of STS course
Product	To impart an unproblematic body of knowledge about the natural world	Empiricist and inductivist; always as common sense	Hierarchical; a transmission-belt from teacher *to* student	Utilitarian
Inquiry	To satisfy curiosity about the way the world is. Sometimes: knowledge for its own sake and the reproduction of practitioner science	A method of enquiry; frequently Popperian	A partnership, though not an equal one	Liberal/humanistic
Relevance	Acquisition of knowledge for the sake of collective liberation and personal development	Problem-solving response to human needs	Collaborative inquiry into matters of agreed concern	Reflexive

Source: Adapted from Table 2 in Judith Hargreaves and Tony Hargreaves, "Some Models of School Science in British Curriculum Projects, and their Implications for STS Teaching at the Secondary Level", *Social Studies of Science*, Vol. 13, No. 4, November 1983.

scientific facts and theories are *social conventions*. This view, which has many "labels" ("epistemological relativist", "social constructivist" and "ethnographic" among them), is taken to be diametrically opposed to *any* "realism", and hence radically challenges orthodox views. Its main achievement is to question the "natural" basis of *scientific* authority, and to relocate it in *social* authority. A similar shift is characteristic of recent studies within the Marxist tradition, summarized in Young's claim that "Science *is* social relations" (see Levidow and Young[12]; Hales[13]). These views obviously have profound implications for science education, which have yet to be developed. I would resist the suggestion that they constitute a "fourth model", however, since I do not see them as comparable to the other three "generative notions": they do not immediately suggest new *patterns* and *aims* for science education. Rather, they present a constant, insistent challenge to the lazy myths embedded in the practice of "normal science education" and hence, perhaps, a catalyst for reflexive innovations.

Conclusion

I have, as requested, discussed some "alternatives" to present patterns of science education, and some of their implications. As the reader will realize, I consider it an open question as to whether such alternatives *should* be "integrated properly into teaching", and also whether they *can* be. The latter doubt hinges on the crucial role of power structures and vested interests, both within education and in society at large, in inhibiting radical changes that are perceived as threatening.

It might be thought that a compromise is possible. Could future science education not consist of a *mixture* of these alternatives, with students moving freely between contexts of differing "texture" and rationale—and hence encountering STS and ethical issues in their appropriate contexts, as a natural part of the whole educational process? I admit both that such a compromise is *possible*, and that students *can* do justice to such a "pluralistic" experience. But I submit that the growth of *any* alternative to the "product" model constitutes a threat to those committed to that model: and, since the latter group is both in the majority and in power, any compromise is likely to be transient and unstable. But this is merely to say that the problem is essentially *political*.

---

12. J. Levidow & B. Young, *Science, Technology and the Labour Process: Marxist Studies*, Vol. 1, Humanities Press and CSE Books, 1981.
13. M. Hales, *Science or Society? The Politics of the Work of Scientists*, Pan Books and Channel 4 TV, 1983.

RELIGION, VALUES
AND SCIENCE EDUCATION

Ian G. Barbour

At the World Council of Churches' conference at MIT in 1979, scientists and theologians explored the relevance of the Christian faith for a world of science-based technology. One of the working groups considered some broad questions on science and education, but it did not examine in detail the structure of the science curriculum.[1] In this paper I will ask in what ways religious beliefs in general and Christian beliefs in particular might be relevant to three aspects of science: (1) scientific theories, (2) priorities in scientific research, and (3) policy choices involving applied science. Then I will explore some implications for the college and university curriculum.

Religion and scientific theories

Religious faith is not directly relevant to the analysis of specific scientific theories. The history of the church's interference in scientific debate since the time of Copernicus and Galileo has led to a justifiable demand for the autonomy of science. Past conflicts have arisen from misunderstandings of the nature of religious assertions, or from misunderstandings of the nature of scientific assertions. Linguistic philosophy has helped us to clarify the differing functions of scientific and religious language, and biblical scholarship has illuminated the historical character of the scriptural record.

Classical theologians from Augustine to Luther held that there are "levels of truth" in scripture and they allowed for the allegorical or metaphorical interpretation of particular passages. In the later Reformation period, biblical literalism was more common, and it has continued among some contemporary evangelical Protestants. But today the Roman Catholic Church and the main-line Protestant denominations are critical of scriptural literalism. For example, the opening chapters of Genesis are usually understood to be an enduring theological affirmation about God's relation to the world, expressed in a story which reflects the limited scientific knowledge of its time. The message is that

---

1. P. Abrecht ed., *Faith and Science in an Unjust World*, Vol. 2, Geneva, World Council of Churches, 1980, chapter 3.

God is sovereign, transcendent and purposeful—a message which excludes pantheism and atheism, but which is compatible with a variety of scientific accounts. The creation story also affirms that the world is orderly, dependable and essentially good. These are basically assertions about every moment in time, not about events distant in time. In such a perspective we can speak of evolution as God's way of creating.[2]

But should we at least welcome the "Big Bang" theory in astronomy as scientific support for the doctrine of creation? In the 1960s, some astronomers favoured the Steady State theory which postulated uniform processes during an infinite span of time and space. However the 1965 discovery of the 3 °K background radiation permeating the universe strongly favours the hypothesis of an explosive expansion from a very dense primordial nucleus some 20 billion years ago. The "Big Bang" theory does seem to resemble the Genesis account in pointing to an initial singularity. But a beginning in time is not an essential component of the doctrine of creation. Thomas Aquinas, for example, maintained that the world's dependence on God would be equally compatible with the idea of an infinite time-span. Moreover, there are astronomers who postulate an oscillating universe in which the universe collapsed into a single massive fireball before the current expansive phase. I would submit that the choice of theories in astrophysics must be made on scientific grounds alone. Theologians do not have a stake in the outcome. It is as difficult for us to imagine that time had a beginning as it is to imagine that time is infinite. And in both cases the scientist leaves two questions unanswered: Why does the world exist at all? Why does it have the structure it has?[3]

Religious faith may of course influence the selection of topics which a scientist or a social group considers most important for research. Moreover, religious, philosophical and cultural assumptions may have some influence on the kinds of concepts or hypotheses which a scientist constructs.[4] Nevertheless, the choice among competing scientific theories must be made by the scientific community alone.

Apart from particular theories, there are in modern science three general characteristics whose philosophical and theological implications might be discussed in some science courses:

1. The interplay of *chance and law* is crucial in many areas of science, from quantum physics to evolutionary theory. The impact of these ideas on human

---

2. I. Barbour, *Issues in Science and Religion*, Englewood Cliffs, NJ, Prentice-Hall, 1966; A.R. Peacocke, *Creation and the World of Science*, Oxford, Clarendon Press, 1979; C. Birch and J. Cobb, *The Liberation of Life*, Cambridge, Cambridge University Press, 1981.

3. E. McMullin, "How Should Cosmology Relate to Theology", *The Sciences and Theology in the Twentieth Century*, A.R. Peacocke ed., Notre Dame, Ind., University of Notre Dame Press, 1981.

4. G. Holton, *Thematic Origins of Scientific Thought*, Cambridge, Mass., Harvard University Press, 1973.

thought during the last century could be considered. The compatibility or incompatibility of chance and law with ideas of purpose and creativity in the universe could be explored.[5]

2. The scientist studies *human beings as a part of nature.* Any claim concerning the uniqueness of humanity must take into account our evolutionary history, our dependence on the non-human world, and the ways in which we are similar to other forms of life as well as different from them.

3. Science is often *reductionistic.* We try to understand the behaviour of complex wholes in terms of the behaviour of their parts. Of course, there are also theories and concepts which are applicable only to the higher levels of organization of organisms or ecosystems. Moreover, the mechanistic concepts of Newtonian science have often been replaced or supplemented by more dynamic and holistic concepts involving fields, ecosystems, and the relationship of the observer to that which is observed.

The study of science often seems to have a materialistic impact on the outlook of students. This may be partly the result of preoccupation with science to the exclusion of other areas of interest and experience. It may also be a product of the attempt to rely exclusively on the methods of science. The mechanistic concepts prominent in many sciences since Newton have sometimes been extended into a mechanistic and deterministic world-view. Such an interpretation neglects the selective character of scientific constructs and extends a limited theory into a total metaphysical system. Today we can point to the importance of social, aesthetic and religious experience and the need to go beyond science in gaining a more holistic understanding of the world. Both the churches and the university have a responsibility to help the science student see the findings of science within a larger framework of meaning.

The science teacher can note the temptation to take a methodological assumption which is fruitful at a certain period in the history of science and extend it into a universal metaphysics concerning the nature of reality. Science teachers can convey to students some sense of the limitations of the methods of science and some humility concerning the tentative and selective character of scientific theories. I will consider later how this might be done in particular courses.

Priorities in scientific research
The directions in which scientific research is pursued are influenced by the goals of the institutions which support science. The selection of problems for research in applied science is largely determined by the economic interests of industry and the political goals of government, and this in turn exerts indirect pressure on the allocation of funds for basic research. In some fields such as molecular biology and solid-state physics the distinction between pure and

---

5. Barbour, *op. cit.*

applied science is often blurred, and the time between scientific discovery and practical application is very short. Again, basic medical research has been directed disproportionately towards the diseases of the affluent, to the neglect of tropical diseases and chronic illness affecting a larger fraction of mankind.

At the World Council of Churches' conference there was some disagreement concerning the influence of political and economic interests on basic research. Prof. Hanbury Brown defended the ideal of the objective, value-free scientist dedicated to the pursuit of truth, though he acknowledged the increasing industrialization of applied science. He argued that in basic research an autonomous scientific community should be guided only by the internal logic of science itself. By contrast, Rubem Alves and Jerry Ravetz held that priorities in scientific research are determined in practice by the goals of the institutions which support it. Even in the academic world, the availability of industrial contracts or government grants often dominates the choice of research topics. One out of three scientists and engineers alive today is directly or indirectly involved in military research, according to United Nations figures.[6]

One can find examples which fit each of these models. Astrophysics and astronomy, for instance, are relatively free from industrial and political influence. But a considerable portion of academic research in molecular biology is funded by corporations interested in potential commercialization. I would guess that most forms of basic research fall between these extremes. The typical research scientist is strongly motivated by intellectual curiosity and the desire to gain the respect of the scientific community, but the constraints introduced by the need for financial support cannot be ignored.

The biblical tradition cannot provide any simple answer to this debate. On the one hand, it holds that God as creator is the source of all truth, and that our intellectual capacities are likewise God-given. On the other, it reminds us of the tendency of all persons and all institutions to pursue narrowly conceived goals and to put self-interest ahead of social justice and human welfare. I will suggest that in our work as scientists we need to be more aware of the social context of science, and we need to help our students gain such an awareness.

Policy choices involving applied science

Turning from pure science to applied science and technology, at what points might biblical religion be relevant? There are three broad themes which would affect our response to modern technology:

First, the Bible holds up a distinctive view of *human fulfilment*. It does not minimize the importance of food and shelter and health. From the laws of Deuteronomy and the message of the prophets to the gospels and epistles there are repeated calls for action to alleviate physical suffering, especially among the underprivileged. Active response to the neighbour in need is the basis on

---

6. R. Shinn ed., *Faith and Science in an Unjust World*, Vol. 1, Geneva, World Council of Churches, 1980.

which we will be judged: "For I was hungry and you gave me food . . . I was naked and you clothed me, I was sick and you visited me" (Matt. 25:35). Much of modern technology, especially in agriculture and medicine, can be seen as a response to such physical needs.

But the Bible also insists that "man does not live by bread alone". It points to the dangers of affluence and luxury. It identifies the good life not with material consumption or possessions but with personal existence in community. The God of Israel is interested in the fabric of the community's life and the character of personal interactions. The New Testament speaks of reconciliation between persons. Fulfilment consists of right relationship to God and neighbour. Such concern for personal existence should make us aware of the depersonalizing tendencies of modern industrialism. Respect for human dignity today includes sensitivity to the effects of technology on people and the subtle ways in which persons can be manipulated. In awareness of the sacred and recognition of mystery and human limitations there are correctives to excessive claims for technology. Receptivity and acknowledgment of grace stand in contrast to the attitudes of control and manipulation which a technological society encourages. The Christian tradition cherishes dimensions of human experience which are not accessible to technical reason.

Second, the biblical view of *human nature* combines realism with idealism. Human sinfulness refers not only to the actions of individuals, but also to social institutions. Every group tends to rationalize its own self-interest. The recognition of human fallibility and the abuse of power should make us hesitant to turn over social decisions to technical experts, however well-intentioned. It also might make us more cautious about large-scale systems in which human error or institutional self-interest could have catastrophic consequences. When technology gives us the power to destroy ourselves, humility is a survival need. But the biblical tradition is also idealistic in its vision of creative human potentialities and the possibility of a more just social order. It sees political processes as a vehicle for both the restraint of power and the fight for social justice. It would lead us to try to redirect technology rather than simply to reject it.

Third, religion can be a source of *individual and social change*. At the personal level, the biblical message holds out the possibility of release from guilt and anxiety, liberation from self-centredness, and a life of genuine relatedness and openness when the power of love breaks into our encapsulated lives. Healing, wholeness, and reconciliation can take place between persons, in communities of mutual acceptance, and in the relations between groups. The biblical imagination also has looked to a future kingdom of peace and brotherhood on earth. Today, visions of alternative futures can be a source of hope and renewal. Such a future would involve new definitions of what is necessary to sustain a good life, social patterns in which cooperation replaces competition, and life-styles that avoid the compulsion to consume. The ideal of simplicity can be recovered, not in a spirit of ascetic self-denial, but because global resources are limited—and because there are positive values in a simpler life and sources of satisfaction that are not resource-intensive.

In these three themes the church has a distinctive message for a technological society. Such themes can also contribute to the outlook of the individual science teacher who is a Christian. But I submit that in public discussion of policy choices in a pluralistic culture the ethical issues should be analyzed, not in these theological categories, but in terms of values concerning which Christian and non-Christian can make common cause. Consider the values which were central at the WCC conference: justice, participation and sustainability.

1. *Justice.* Justice has been a major concern of the biblical tradition from the Hebrew prophets to the contemporary church. The gap between rich and poor has been judged in the light of the fundamental equality of all persons before God. Oppression of the poor is condemned both as a violation of human relationships within the community and as a failure in responding to a God of justice and righteousness. But justice has also been prominent in the writings of philosophers since Plato. John Rawls has recently argued that principles of justice can be derived by imagining a social contract between persons who do not know in what social position they will live. Such contractors, he maintains, would allow only those inequalities in the distribution of income and wealth which would maximize the benefits to the least advantaged, since any of them might end up in the worst-off position. As in biblical religion, the treatment of the dispossessed serves as a test case for justice in society.[7] Almost all policy choices concerning technology involve issues of justice in the distribution of costs, benefits and risks.

2. *Participation.* I would argue that we should think of freedom not individualistically as the absence of constraints but socially as the opportunity to participate in the decisions which affect our lives. In biblical terms, participation is both a means of achieving justice and an assertion of individual dignity and responsibility. Philosophers have given much attention to political freedom, democratic forms of government, and civil liberties such as freedom of worship and freedom of speech. The challenge today is to find political mechanisms through which both citizens and experts can contribute to the complex decisions of a technological society. This requires an informed citizenry with access to relevant information and a voice in public decisions about technology. Large-scale centralized technologies accelerate the concentration of economic and political power, whereas most decentralized or "appropriate" technologies are more amenable to community control and local participation.[8]

---

7. J. Rawls, *A Theory of Justice*, Cambridge, Mass., Harvard University Press, 1971.
8. I. Barbour, *Technology, Environment and Human Values*, New York, Praeger, 1980; R. Shinn, *Forced Options*, New York, Harper & Row, 1982.

3. *Sustainability*. Included here are both environmental preservation and resource use as long-term global issues. Many authors have pointed out that the biblical theme of dominion over nature is not a licence for unlimited exploitation but a call to responsible stewardship. The Bible also speaks of obligations to posterity and accountability to a God whose purposes span the generations. The land, for example, is to be held as a trust for future generations. Recently there has been extensive philosophical exploration of environmental ethics, animal rights, and obligations to future generations. From the scientific side, ecologists have made us more aware of the interdependence of the community of life and the far-reaching repercussions of our actions. We have begun to study the carrying capacity of environments and the sustainability of both renewable and non-renewable resources. Through technology we have often been able to offset the depletion of non-renewable resources by discovering new reserves, introducing new extraction techniques, or finding substitutes for scarce materials—but usually at a cost in environmental impact and energy use. Sustainability today entails efficient use, restraining growth in consumption in affluent societies, and facilitating the transition to abundant or renewable resources.[9]

In addition to justice, participation and sustainability, there are other values on which Christians and non-Christians can agree, such as health and safety, employment and economic growth, and world peace. I will suggest how the trade-offs among these values can be considered in specific policy decisions.

The university curriculum

A science curriculum which might be appropriate in one type of college or university might be quite unsuitable in another academic context. I can only give examples of the ways in which the principles I have outlined might be applied in four types of courses. My examples are taken from the United States because I am more familiar with what is being done there.

TECHNICAL SCIENCE AND ENGINEERING

Within standard science and engineering courses there is always great pressure to try to cover a large amount of technical material. Nevertheless it is possible to give students at least some sense of science not just as a body of information but as a process. Reference to the history of science and the social context of scientific research can give some picture of the scientific enterprise, going beyond the memorization of formulas or the mastery of principles. Sometimes this can be done through more detailed case studies of the development of a particular theory or technological application, even if other theories or applications have to be treated more briefly.

---

9. R. Nelson, *Science and Our Troubled Conscience*, Philadelphia, Fortress Press, 1980; L. Brown, *Building a Sustainable Society*, New York, W.W. Norton, 1981.

In discussing a scientific theory such as Newtonian mechanics, quantum theory, or Darwin's theory of evolution, it would be appropriate in some courses to discuss the impact of the theory on human thought outside of science. Similarly a course on a technology such as computers could look at its social impacts. Moreover, discussion of interactions in both directions between science and society is important for non-scientists seeking an understanding of science. We should note also the influence of the example set by the scientist's own involvement in public activities, such as writing articles designed to inform the public, serving on advisory panels, or appearing as an expert witness at legislative or regulatory hearings or court trials (at the local, regional or national level). There are many environmental, consumer and citizens' organizations in which scientists can work with public-interest groups on educational or legislative projects.

PROFESSIONAL ETHICS

The 1970s saw a rapid growth in the study of medical ethics and bio-ethics both in pre-medical education and in medical schools. Courses in environmental ethics were also developed, with a substantial literature and journals from which to draw. A number of universities have introduced offerings in engineering ethics, and some excellent teaching materials and case studies have appeared. Courses on ethical issues in science are less common but could be expanded.[10]

Here are some of the types of questions which can be raised in such courses:[11]

— What ethical issues arise in choice of a research topic, research on animal or human subjects, allocation of credit, or relationships to subordinates or superiors in scientific work?
— Under what circumstances does the scientist's social responsibility extend beyond the pursuit of truth to include consideration of possible consequences of his or her work, insofar as they can be foreseen? How can such responsibility be most effectively expressed?
— How can scientists balance loyalties to their employers, their profession, and the public in calling attention to potential risks arising from their work?

---

10. R. Baum, *Ethics and Engineering Curricula*, Hastings-on-Hudson, NY, The Hastings Center, 1980; R. Flores and R. Baum, *Ethical Problems in Engineering*, Troy, NY, Rensselaer Polytechnic Institute, 1980; J.H. Schaub and K. Pavlovic, *Engineering Professionalism and Ethics*, New York, John Wiley, 1982; S. Unger, *Controlling Technology: Ethics and the Responsible Engineer*, New York, Holt, Rinehart & Winston, 1983.
11. G. Holton and R. Morrison, *The Limits of Scientific Inquiry*, New York, W.W. Norton, 1979; A. Flores and D. Taber, "Annotated Bibliography on Professional Ethics of Scientists", *Research in Philosophy and Technology*, Vol. 5, 1982; T. Segerstedt ed., *Ethics for Science Policy*, New York, Pergamon, 1980.

What role can professional societies play in protecting members who are penalized for speaking out on such issues?
— Are codes of professional ethics an effective instrument for protecting the interests of the public as well as the interests of the profession?
— At what point is the increasingly competitive nature of research detrimental to either personal integrity or scientific progress (secrecy, patentability, priority rivalry, grantsmanship, publicity through the media, etc.)?
— What personal or procedural guidelines address the problem of the scientist as adviser or expert witness on panels or at public hearings (scientific uncertainty, conflicting expertise, disciplinary or institutional biases, etc.)?
— In a time of increasing cooperation between industry and academia in fields such as molecular biology and computer science, what contractual arrangements will protect legitimate intellectual and financial interests of both parties?
— What institutional procedures offer promise of reconciling freedom of scientific inquiry with the demand for greater accountability in science? How should priorities in allocation of government research funds be established?
— What forms of decision-making allow most suitably for both technical expertise and democratic participation in policy decisions?

In discussing such questions, the teaching objective is not to promote a particular answer but to encourage the recognition of ethical issues and the ability to analyze them. In order to avoid indoctrination it is helpful to examine diverse views in particular cases in which scientists have confronted moral dilemmas on the job or in their public activity. The student must engage in critical thinking and moral reasoning in order to develop some capacity for judgment which could carry over to future life. This will require the science teacher to do some serious study in ethics or to work closely with a philosopher or theologian interested in ethical theory and application.

SCIENCE, TECHNOLOGY AND SOCIETY
An important contribution to the education of both future scientists and non-scientists can be made by faculties in the humanities and social sciences. Philosophy of science is a well established field and there is an emerging literature in the philosophy of technology. Some theological faculties and departments of religion offer courses on science and religion or on technology and ethics, and others should be encouraged to do so.

History of science and history of technology are recognized specialties among historians. In many universities courses are now being offered in the sociology of science. All of these fields throw light on science as a process and on the social context of science and its social impacts.

There are professional societies and journals which provide for the exchange of ideas in all of these areas. Among the journals started in recent years are

Social Studies of Science; Science, Technology and Human Values; and *Bulletin of Science, Technology and Society*. Some excellent teaching materials have been prepared under the leadership of W.F. Williams of the University of Leeds in the project known as SISCON (Science in a Social Context). There are a number of programmes at American universities and technical schools offering groups of related courses, and in many cases graduate degrees, in science, technology and society. Among these are programmes at Cornell University, Washington University in St Louis, MIT, Virginia Polytechnic and Rensselaer Polytechnic. In all these programmes scientists are active participants, along with philosophers, historians and sociologists.[12]

Science, technology and public policy

I believe that the most promising way to raise ethical issues concerning applied science and technology is to develop courses dealing with specific public issues such as energy policy, environmental policy, mineral policy, food and agricultural policy, or nuclear weapons policy. By focusing on particular past, present and future policy decisions, the scientific, economic, political and ethical dimensions and their inter-relations can be brought out. In case studies of policy analysis the relevance of justice, participation, sustainability and other values mentioned earlier will be evident. There will be opportunity for systematic ethical reasoning in real-life situations involving current legislation, resource planning and our choices as citizens, consumers and scientists. Resource policies typically require consideration of interactions between technology, the environment, and economic and political institutions.[13]

The students in such interdisciplinary courses will be specializing in science, engineering, economics, government and political science, law, and a variety of other fields. Where possible the course should be team-taught or should allow participation by colleagues in other fields. Here again it is desirable for scientists to gain some competence in ethics and politics. This is not easy to do because the academic reward structure is so highly departmentalized. Promotions and tenure are based primarily on specialized research, while teaching, particularly in interdisciplinary areas, receives little recognition. We should encourage academic institutions to give more formal support to such policy-related courses and to public policy programmes in which these issues so crucial to the future of the world can receive attention from both students and professors.

---

12. A. Teich ed., *Technology and Man's Future*, 3rd ed., New York, St Martin's Press, 1981; S. Lakoff ed., *Science and Ethical Responsibility*, Reading, Mass., Addison–Wesley, 1980.
13. T. Kuhn and A. Porter, *Science, Technology and National Policy*; M. Krantzberg ed., *Ethics in an Age of Pervasive Technology*, Boulder, Colo., Westview, 1980. See also I. Barbour, *Technology, Environment and Human Values, op. cit.*

VALUES, RESPONSIBILITIES AND COMMITMENTS IN THE TEACHING OF SCIENCE

Charles Birch

There are two major defects in the teaching of science today. One is its failure to lead to any adequate philosophical model of the world around us and within us. The other is the failure of science to invest its facts with values, with the consequence that it appears to be ethically and morally detached. These two defects in the teaching of science are inter-related and are at the heart of the problem of relating science and faith.

Science as it is taught in schools and colleges and universities in the western world is largely science detached from values. Attempts are made to restore values in some interdisciplinary courses such as the history and philosophy of science or science technology and society, but these can hardly get at the root of the problem when the basic teaching in physics, chemistry and biology lead to a dominant model of the universe—its atoms, cells and living organisms including humans—as machines.

I was recently invited by the one time Archbishop of Melbourne, Sir Frank Woods, to address science teachers in church schools in the State of Victoria on the relation between science and faith. The Archbishop was moved to do something because on his rounds of church schools he was often told by students that science has made religion old hat. Science deals with facts, religion with non-facts. There was no room for faith in a world of science and technology. Why, he asked, did the teaching of science in schools lead to this sort of conclusion? Of course, he might also have asked, and no doubt did, why the teaching of religion in schools seemed to reinforce the gap between science and faith. The discussion we had on that occasion with science teachers, including quite a number of school principals, showed that they were deeply disturbed about the failure of their teaching to bridge the gap between science and faith, or science and the values that faith seeks to promote. They felt deeply the need for resource materials both for themselves and for their classes. The first decision of the group was to find or produce such materials.

The failure of science to bestow values on the facts with which it deals has far-reaching effects. It is a major cause of the malaise of the western world with its heavily conditioned atmosphere of secularism and materialism. Mass media press this atmosphere into every life and every home with the result that widespread beliefs appear to be axiomatic when they are no more than the conditioned assumptions of this generation.

Human beings need meaning in addition to information. This need for meaning, purpose and fulfilment lies deeply in our nature. It is subverted when science becomes detached from values. When science leads to an image of the universe and all that is in it, including humans, as contrivance or machine, it has excluded values from information. When science operates without a sensitive conscience about the influence of its discoveries on the life of the world, it has excluded values from information. This omission finds expression in the yearnings of those who feel lost in an age committed to technological progress and which seeks solutions to human problems in technology and economics. Our problems are neither primarily technological nor economic. They are conceptual. The proliferation of cults and sects and movements such as creationism in our time are reactions to the loss of a sense of our place in the cosmic scheme of things. They are symptoms of a disease.

The substantialist prejudice

The dominant model of the world derived from science, through what I believe is a misunderstanding of science, is a counterfeit model. It is the model of the world and all that is in it as contrivance or factory. It is the clockwork universe that produces a clockwork society. Likewise the alternative we are so often offered, namely a dichotomy between matter and mind, nature and God, science and faith is also counterfeit. Yet this is a dominant model in much of traditional religion in the West today. It is unable to deal with the fundamental questions that come from either science or faith. It arose historically as a sort of gentleman's agreement between science and faith. It is commonly stated in the gentlemanly form—science deals with how and religion deals with why. This is just another way of keeping science and faith apart. Yet both science and faith are concerned with what's what in the world. From affirmations made about that world all sorts of ethical and moral issues flow. If we get the picture of the world wrong we get a warped picture of life. As Abraham Maslow said: "To him who has only a hammer the whole world looks like a nail."

In the dominant mechanistic or substantialist paradigm the view of entities, be they atoms or humans, is that they are independent of other entities. That is the definition of a machine. It is subject only to the law of mechanics. It has only external relations such as the energy that is fed into it. This is the notion of substance. A substance has only external relations. We are prejudiced to think of all entities as self-contained in this way, even cells and humans. It is the substantialist prejudice. So we attempt to analyze entities, be they rocks or stars or humans into other entities which we think are even more substantial and enduring than they are. This is the classical notion of Democritus' atoms that are indivisible and unchanging.

Our society operates out of a profound error that is destroying much that is worthwhile in ourselves and in the world when it opts for the substantialist prejudice. Consider what it does in our universities. The substantialist prejudice leads to a substantialist view of the disciplines. We separate knowledge into disciplines, each being a substance in its own right. When you get a discipline you get a department. The function of a department is to produce experts in that discipline. Sometimes experts cross boundaries. Mostly they don't. Heidegger said science doesn't think. By this he meant scientists do not cross boundaries. They don't cross disciplines. There is a difference between an expert and a thinker. The thinker crosses boundaries. The expert sees knowledge as a jigsaw puzzle. You work on your bit and I work on mine. Then we put the pieces together to get the picture of the truth. The general idea has been that if society has well-trained experts in all the disciplines the experts would guide us in the truth and to right action. It hasn't worked out that way. What went wrong?

Knowledge is not like the blocks in a jigsaw puzzle. The title of Arthur Koestler's last book is *Bricks to Babel*. In it he wrote: "We seem to be compelled to shape facts and data as we know them into hard bricks and stick them together with the slime of our theories and beliefs." The result—a tower of Babel. That is why Bernard Shaw, in *The Doctor's Dilemma*, said: "The professions are all a conspiracy against the laity." The experts are always wrong.

Theology has some resistance against being brought into this orbit. But by degrees it has retreated into a discipline in its own right unrelated to the rest of the world. But to restrict the province in which you think is to run counter to Christian self-understanding. In traditional (but not orthodox) Christian teaching, God is defined as substance—independent and unrelated to anything else. Perfection is supposed to have that kind of character. But if the world is dependent upon God and if God is influenced by the world then God is not a substance. Theology and much of Christian thought retreated from this view and cut God off from the world and the world from God. So we are given concepts of God that are irrelevent to the world. That is both profoundly unbiblical and profoundly incorrect.

The substantialist universe and God

The great success of the scientific method is largely due to the methodology of mechanism. Science investigates the universe and its parts as if the universe and its parts were machines or substances. Human physiology never got off the ground until it began to investigate the heart as a pump and the limbs as levers. It is one thing to investigate entities such as living organisms as if they were machines (methodological mechanism). It is quite another to assert that these entities *are* machines (metaphysical mechanism).

Each age of science has tended to present us with a remodelled mechanical picture of the universe. In the sixteenth century Copernicus gave us a picture of the cosmos as an ordered system of celestial bodies. This system fell into Galileo's lap. All is mathematics. Only that which is measurable is real. Galileo argued that God holds the planets in position in their orbits as they sing the music of the spheres in praise of him. Then came Newton telling us that the same principle that accounts for the fall of the apple also holds the planets in place—the principle of gravitation. All that was left for God to do was to return occasionally to put the planets in phase, much as a spaceship receives correcting messages from its earth stations.

Hence we get the picture of the universe as a complex machine or contrivance. God the prime mover becomes the occasional mechanic returning to tune the mechanism. But the comets were still a problem. They didn't seem to obey any laws. From time immemorial they were held as portents of God's intervention into the world. The predicted return of Halley's comet in 1759 changed all that. Now even the comets came within the ordered system of Newtonian mechanics. So when Laplace explained his system of celestial mechanics to Napoleon, the emperor asked: "And where does God come into your scheme?" Laplace replied: "Sire, I have no need of that hypothesis." There was no place for God in a universe that was completely mechanical in its nature. All was to be interpreted in terms of the size and shape and disposition of building blocks called atoms. Besides them nothing else exists. Laplace claimed that if he knew the number, size and forces between the atoms he could predict the future of the universe. This is what Whitehead[1] was to call the "billiard-ball universe".

By the middle of the nineteenth century God was pushed outside the universe except for the plants and animals. They were the direct result of his designing hand. They were the products of blueprints on the creator's drawing board. The great eighteenth century naturalists like John Ray thought so. So did Archdeacon Paley whose *Natural Theology* was required reading until this century for all students at Cambridge University. This was the watch-maker analogy of the relation of the creatures to God, an image which was used at least as far back as the fourteenth century by a French bishop Nicole Oresme.[2] And so thought Charles Darwin who, as a student at Cambridge, was greatly impressed by Paley's argument. But eventually his voyage of discovery on the "Beagle" was to change all that. The designer God becomes replaced by natural selection of chance variations. God is pushed out of the direct ordering of nature back into the origin of life.

Darwinism clashed with nineteenth century deism at three points. According to Darwin:

—Nature is and always has been in process of being made. It was not made once and for all in perfection, but is incomplete.

---

1. A.N. Whitehead, *Science and the Modern World,* New York, Macmillan, 1926.
2. Lyn White, "Christianity and Nature", *Pacific Theological Review*, 7, 1975, pp. 6–11.

—The processes of change involve chance in the form of chance variations on which natural selection acts. These chance changes were later to be called mutations.

—Natural selection depends upon a struggle for existence. Instead of nature being benign it is, in Tennyson's phrase, "red in tooth and claw". Huxley said it was a "gigantic gladiatorial show".

How then can we square the fact of an uncompleted creation, the existence of misfits, the element of chance and struggle with a loving God who made it once and for all perfect? Bertrand Russell said that if he were granted omnipotence and millions of years in which to experiment, he thought he could have done a better job and a more direct one. It is difficult, he said, not to feel as the boy did after being taught the alphabet, that it was not worth going through so much to get so little.

So Darwin and Huxley and many others called themselves agnostics. Darwin himself said: "I cannot see the universe as a result of chance and yet I cannot see each separate being as a result of design. I am in a complete muddle." Others like the marine biologist, Philip Gosse, refused to accept the new knowledge and remained deists. Yet a third response was typified by Charles Kingsley, the English vicar and novelist, who said: "Now that they have got rid of an interfering God, master magician as I call it, they have to choose between the absolute empire of accident and a living immanent ever-working God." The "doctrine of divine carpentry", as Canon Charles Raven called the doctrine of deism, could now give way to a more credible concept of divine creativity.

Kingsley and Raven in their different ways were arguing against the substance notion of the world and the substance notion of God outside the world. But there was nothing new about this. In orthodox Christian teaching God was not substance unrelated to the universe. God was sustainer of the universe in the sense that without God the world would collapse. The universe was not a self-sufficient machine. Over the centuries science persuaded theology that the hypothesis of God sustaining the world in some sense was not necessary for science. So for theology the world became independent of God's activity, except for occasional interventions in the form of floods or plagues. The world can get along without God. It is a common view amongst Christians today. It has an interesting corollary. If the world can get along without God then God can get along without the world. Both are wrong.

Two ways of interpreting the world around us and the world within us

There are two ways of trying to understand the world around us. One is to reduce it to as near to nothing as possible (such as the atoms or their parts), and then try to build up a world from these "building blocks". The movement is from Atom to Eve. But that supposes that atoms in living cells are the same as atoms not in living cells, and that atoms in human brains are the same as atoms not in human brains. If atoms are the same everywhere independent of the environment in which they find themselves, then if you construct a world from them of course you get a machine. This is profoundly wrong.

But supposing we start our journey of understanding at the other end; not with the classical atoms of the physicist but with that collection of atoms which constitutes us and particularly that constellation of atoms which constitutes that most complex of all arrangements of atoms that exist so far as we know, human brains, and from them work backwards—what then? We shall reach quite another conclusion. The first way is to interpret the higher in terms of the lower levels and organization. The second way is to interpret the lower in terms of the higher. I do not know the great Amazon river by studying it only at its sources in rivulets in the Andes. I have to see what the Amazon becomes at its mouth. Likewise I cannot know what atoms or electrons are by looking at them after dissecting the universe down to its building blocks. I have to see what they become. They become human brains with human thoughts and feelings. Now a universe that produces human beings is a different universe from one that could not do so. It is a humanizing universe. Norman Mailer said: "If the universe is a lock then the key to that lock is not a measure but a metaphor." The metaphor is personality. Personality, not classical physics, is the key to the universe.

The basic principle I am proposing is that we understand what is not ourselves by analogy with what we know ourselves to be. The principle is stated clearly in the prologue to St John's Gospel and in the first two chapters of Genesis. There the answer to the question what is man is given not in terms of substance but in terms of relationships that are personal. There are no substances. There are experiences. I am what I am by virture of my relationships, not the ones that push and pull me hither and thither but the internal relations that make me feel elated, depressed, sad, joyous and so on. These relations have nothing to do with the laws of mechanics. The idea of internal relations is one that is constitutive of the character or even the very existence of the entity.

Instead of the world as made of substances, let us think of it as made of events. The hydrogen atom is an event depicted by a positive charge surrounded by a negative charge. Stop the electronic event and there is no hydrogen atom. Entities such as atoms and cells and humans take account of their environment internally. They are subjects. That is to say they have subjective experience. Now of course that aspect is greatly attenuated in the inanimate world so that most people tend to rule out the possibility that it is a part of nature there at all. But we do usually acknowledge that human beings and our pets at least are subjects. Subjects are not primarily means but are ends in themselves. We respect them for what they are in themselves, for themselves and for God. Science, whatever its virtues, is at best a language of objects and not subjects. Sociology and psychology should remember that!

What I am suggesting is that not only humans are subjects that are characterized by internal relations, but there are entities all down the line from humans back to atoms and electrons taking account of their environment internally. They are what they are by virtue of the internal relations established in different environments. A sodium atom in the molecule sodium chloride is not the same as a sodium atom not in sodium chloride. When it is alone the sodium atom has peculiar metallic properties. And when alone the chlorine atom has gaseous properties. But in the appropriate combination in the sodium chloride molecule new qualities emerge which we did not appreciate before, such as the quality of saltiness. We know more about the atoms chlorine and sodium when we know about them in the particular relations in which they exist together in sodium chloride. Likewise with all atoms in all their different possible combinations, such for example as in human brains. So too cells in brains are different from cells not in brains. Humans in this particular relationship are different from humans in that particular relationship. This is an ecological model of existence as opposed to the substance model.[3]

What have modern physics and biology to say to the ecological model?
    In physics the notion of substance received a profound blow when physics began to more towards an ecological model. The modern physicist still talks about fundamental particles. Not one of them believes in particles any more. Neither electrons nor protons nor any other such entity is a particle. We may have an image of a particle but that is our construction. The hunt for the elusive quark will not end up in the discovery of a lump of stuff of some sort. The physicist's particles (for want of a better word) are not things but events.
    Prof. David Bohm, a quantum physicist in London University, thinks that physics has got itself into a hopeless mess with substance thinking with its images of waves and particles, both of which are substance notions. He asks us to give up altogether the notion that the world is constituted of basic objects or building blocks. To advance, he says, we must think of the implicate order which is the order due to internal relations. We have to think inside out. By analogy the explicate order is the picture on the television screen. The implicate order in this example is the unseen message that goes through space to make the picture. The physicist's view of matter has been changing so much that Niels Bohr said of Heisenberg's theory: "This is a mad theory. The question is whether it is mad enough to be true."
    Another analogy Bohm uses is the hologram. A regular camera gives us a point picture of the object. Cut the negative in half and you get half the picture. In the hologram when you do the corresponding manipulation you get not half the picture but the whole in attenuated form. It is a holistic way of perceiving an object.

---

3. C. Birch & J.B. Cobb, *The Liberation of Life: From Cell to Community*, Cambridge University Press, 1981.

In biology Pribram uses the same holographic model for the occipital lobe of the brain. This is the part of the brain that registers stimuli from the retina of the eye. Pribram tells us that each cell in the lobe registers the whole image from the eye rather than each cell registering one part of a mosaic. Each cell registers all the relations. Many cells together presumably give the clearest picture. It is not parts, but relationships of the whole that each cell registers.

In genetics we used to speak of Mendelian genetics as particulate genetics. This was because Mendelian genetics was to be contrasted with what went before, namely "blending inheritance". Characters were thought to blend in inheritance. Mendel showed that they did not blend. They retained their integrity. It looked as though particles were inherited. But the gene is no longer thought of as a particle. We say it is a DNA molecule. But how one bit of the molecule expresses itself depends very much on the environment, that is to say on the rest of the molecule and the other genes that are part of its environment. The modern concept of the gene is an ecological one. The gene is more like an organism than like a substance. And so we could add to the story with the view of other biologists who have come to an ecological model of the organism such as C.H. Waddington, Sewall Wright, J.Z. Young and Alister Hardy.

Religious questions

As soon as you break out of the substance paradigm religious questions become important. This is true of each scientist I have mentioned. Substance thinking has been blocking the healthy relation between science and religion. Science has its images of the universe as bits of stuff. Religion has its images of God as substance. We have a substance model of God whenever we conceive of God as independent of other entities in the universe, and whenever we conceive the universe as independent of God. In the ecological model the world is dependent upon God in internal relationships and God is dependent upon the world. How?

The paradigm for the model of the world as dependent upon God is the human person. Man takes account of his environment through internal relations and is transformed by them. This is creative good acting in human life. The source of creative good is God. An analogous influence works within the life of the chimpanzee or the cat or the amoeba and molecules and atoms too. In the ecological model they are sustained through their internal relations. All are subjects which experience or feel in some way, attenuated though this is, no doubt, at the electron level. At each level we recognize internal relations, feelings, perception, freedom, transcendence. The alternative is to believe that at some point in cosmic evolution mind and consciousness were produced from no mind. In the ecological model all are organisms. As A.N. Whitehead has said biology studies the larger organisms and physics studies the smaller organisms. Concerning the question of whether or not the creation experiences, there are three possibilities:

—Matter never experiences, not even the matter in man. This is materialism.

—Matter sometimes experiences, this is matter in man. This is dualism.
—Matter always experiences. This is mentalism or the ecological model.

The universe is a happening of happenings. Stop the happenings and the universe collapses. God is necessary for the world. God is not the world and the world is not God. God is not before all creation but with all creation. The world includes God and God perfects the world. There is no world apart from God.

The aspect of God wherein God sustains the world and lures it to richer experience is what Whitehead calls the primordial nature of God. God's action is not one of coercion but persuasion. God is not the exercise of absolute power. Is God then not omnipotent? If by omnipotence is meant ability to bring about events without relationship to the conditions, then certainly God is not omnipotent. God did not prevent the holocaust. Nor will God prevent the button of nuclear war from being pushed. At every level of the world God operates by persuasive love. God "lures" the creation.

The order of the universe

There are two sorts of ordering process. One is the order produced by a dictator. The other is order through persuasion. The order of "divine carpentry" is the order of a dictatorship. Order in the ecological model is anarchy tamed. Consider the order in a lecture theatre full of people intently listening and responding to a lecturer. The potentiality for disorder there is immense. But the listeners are tamed by their own desire to make the experience a creative one for themselves and others. The order of the universe is of that sort. God is a democrat. But it is not God alone who acts in the world. Every individual acts. There is no single producer. But too many cooks spoil the broth. Multiplicative creativity explains partial disorder. Yet there needs to be a coordinator. A central cosmological problem remained unresolved until this principle became clear.

Cosmic evolution is the successive concrete realization in the world of that which has always been potentially possible from the foundations of the universe. But the possible becomes concrete only in the fullness of time. There is a time and place for every happening. Atoms have to come before cells and so on. In the fullness of time human life appeared. In the fullness of time the life of Jesus became a concrete reality. But in a real sense that possibility was there from the beginning, as is said in the prologue to St John's Gospel.

God as dependent upon the world

In this primordial nature God lures the world to higher levels of transcendence. The creation becomes more aware of God. But God also reacts to the world as it is created. God not only gives but God responds. God is different because of the creation. God without a world is different from God with a world. In the ecological model of God, as the world is created and its evolving entities grow in richness of experience so too does God experience the world. This is what Whitehead calls the consequent nature of God, the nature of God consequent upon creation. Nothing of value is lost. All is saved in the experience and memory of God. Not a sparrow falls to the ground without God knowing.

Even the life of the sparrow has some significance and value to God. Not the merest puff of existence is without some significance to God. In this way God includes the world.

I am asked whether the ecological God is personal. This is a question we must face. However, we need to be careful in using the word person. The image of person is bound up with the substantialist idea of a person as self-contained. It is not a biblical word. It came into theology with the doctrine of the Trinity which tried to put together ideas about God, the world and people. But in the sense that God is involved in my personal being and in yours and all of us are involved in God's being, God is personal, very much so.

Science education

John Ziman[4] blames science education for teaching naive materialism, primitive positivism and complacent technocracy. This is because science education is largely committed to "conventional valid science". This is the science expounded in textbooks and in formal lectures. It is the information you need if you are to build bridges and nuclear power plants or to cure diseases. It is the science behind the technological society. By subordinating to this the contents of every textbook, the message of every lecture and lesson and the demands of every laboratory exercise and examination we neglect our wider educational responsibilities. Conventional valid science eschews fuzzy edges and difficult problems and gives the impression of certainty and rigour to the content of all scientific knowledge. Its images are the images of substance. So it also attempts to be value free. Science education is carried out as if the history, philosophy, sociology and economic aspects of life are unworthy of attention by a serious teacher of dutiful pupils. It finds expression in technological optimism that all things are technically possible and that technology is therefore the solution to all our ills.

Ziman's prescription for change is the development of courses in science, technology and society (STS) in the curricula of schools, colleges and universities. Such courses already exist in quite a number of universities and colleges. But is this enough? What is basically needed is a fundamental change in the mind-set of teachers of science at all levels so that methodological mechanism does not automatically lead to metaphysical mechanism explicit or implied. There needs to be a greater openness to alternative models that are able to incorporate values and other intangibles. I have suggested one such model.

---

4. *Teaching and Learning about Science and Society*, Cambridge University Press, 1980.

There is need also for greater consciousness of the responsibility of the scientist to the society he inevitably helps to create. Shinn[5] emphasizes a distinction between information and commitment. We need lots of information about energy and other resources, for example, if we are to make judgments as to the wisest use of these things. But our judgment will also depend upon our commitments which have to do with values. Commitments guide us in the way we use information. Information and commitments enrich each other. Commitments also provide motivation that produces information. Alternative areas remain unexplored because of lack of basic commitments. Shinn puts the relationship this way: faith without science is silent, science without faith is aimless.[6]

No *deus ex machina* will rescue us from our follies. An ecological view of the world spelt out in detail with information and with an ecological commitment behind it may help to save us.

5. Roger L. Shinn, *Forced Options: Social Decisions for the 21st Century*, San Francisco, Harper & Row, 1982, p. 229.
6. *Ibid.*, p. 226.

MORAL DEVELOPMENT AND EDUCATION

Gerhard Portele

Introduction to Kohlberg's theory on moral development and moral education

The starting point of Kohlberg's theory[1] is Piaget's model for the stages of child development. This shows that development from early childhood onwards is not constant, but occurs in definable stages. Kohlberg calls this the cognitive-developmental approach.

In Piaget's model, the change from one stage to the next is dependent upon a person's interaction with the environment. In each individual personality there is a cognitive system, a stage of logical reasoning or intelligence which allows it to cope with its environment. This cognitive system is in a certain state of equilibrium, but when this state of equilibrium is lost, then the person changes the cognitive system to assimilate and accommodate himself or herself once more into the environment, thus attaining again a cognitive system in equilibrium.

The moral system develops in a one-to-one parallel relationship with the cognitive system. Kohlberg goes as far as to say that moral reasoning *depends* on logical reasoning. There are six stages in moral development. A person moves from stage to stage only in an ascending order and always one stage at a time, although not necessarily reaching the final stage(s) in moral development. The six moral stages can be divided into three major levels: the pre-conventional (stages 1 and 2), the conventional (stages 3 and 4) and the post-conventional (stages 5 and 6). The term "conventional" means conforming to the rules, expectations and conventions of society. Thus the pre-conventional moral level includes most children under nine, some adolescents and adult criminal offenders. The conventional level is that of most adolescents and adults. The post-conventional level is reached only by a minority of adults, usually after the age of 20; someone at this level basically accepts society's

---

1. L. Kohlberg, "Stage and Sequence: the Cognitive Development Approach to Socialization", in D.A. Goslin, *Handbook of Socialization. Theory and Research*, Chicago, 1969.

rules, but this acceptance is based on an understanding of the general underlying moral principles.

Stages 3–6 are the relevant stages for higher education:

Stage 3: "Good boy, good girl": This means living up to what is expected of a person in his/her particular role in society, as a son, brother or a friend for instance. "Being good" means having good motives, showing concern about others, and also showing trust, loyalty, respect and gratitude.

Stage 4: "Law and order": This is the fulfilling of the duties to which a person has agreed. Laws should be upheld except in extreme cases where they conflict with other fixed social duties. It also includes contributing to society.

Stage 5: "Social contract, utility and individual rights": This is to be aware of differing values and opinions, and to understand that most values and rules are relative to a particular group. These rules should be upheld, both in the interest of impartiality and because they constitute the social contract. However non-relative values such as life and liberty should be upheld regardless of majority opinion.

Stage 6: "Universal ethical principles": This means to follow self-chosen ethical principles. Particular laws or social agreements are usually valid because they rest on such principles. When laws violate these principles, then a person acts in accordance with the principles. Principles are universal principles of justice: equality of human rights and respect for the dignity of human beings as individual persons.

A central question on Kohlberg's theory is: what is the relation between moral reasoning and moral behaviour? To identify the developmental stage of a person's moral reasoning, Kohlberg and his associates devised a sophisticated system of standardized scoring. In that system only the form and structure of moral *reasoning* are relevant for the identification of the moral stage. Therefore it is possible that two people in the same stage of moral reasoning make entirely different moral *decisions*. The moral stage is related both to cognitive advance and moral behaviour, but our identification of the moral stage must be based on moral reasoning alone.

In the last years Kohlberg's interest changed from theory to practice. The most important projects, I guess, are the "Intervention in a Prison for Females" and—even more important—"The Cambridge Cluster School. Experiment", where Kohlberg and his co-workers founded the "Just Community School". All I can do here is to cite the principles of the Just Community School.

1. The governance of the school should be one of participatory democracy with students and teachers having equal rights. This implies: (a) rules should not be provided in advance, but made through establishing a social contract between teachers and students, and (b) all major issues of school governance, rules and policy should be made in a (weekly) community or town meeting.

2. The governance structure and community meetings should stress solutions to issues through considerations of fairness and morality.
3. The curriculum or academic classes of the school (especially social studies) should involve developmental moral discussion and should stress basic understanding of concepts of democracy, law and justice. Classroom discussions on morality, law and democracy should be integrated with the real life decisions and policies of the small school community meetings and with the school's relation to the larger school system and society.

The reason for this is very simple:

1. You can only learn to behave morally if you can take responsibility—therefore the community, even the school, must be based on democracy.
2. You can learn moral behaviour only in a just and fair environment.
3. By creating cognitive moral conflicts through discussion of moral and personal dilemmas and by exposure to the next higher stage of moral reasoning you can reach another stage in moral development. Therefore discussion of cognitive moral conflicts has to be part of the curriculum, but that alone is not enough for moral development. It is also necessary to give those who should be educated responsibility for their behaviour in a democratic institution and to create a just and fair community. This is also true for institutions of higher education.

Problems with Kohlberg's theory and subsequent research

Behaviour is a function of personality and environment. Personality consists of at least three systems—the motivational, the cognitive and the moral system. Hence, every action is preceded, either consciously or more often unconsciously, by three main questions:

1. What does a person want? What is his/her motivation?
2. Is the action a realistic possibility?
3. Is it a legitimate action? Is he/she allowed/obliged to act?

Kohlberg only considers the final question. Most actions are *selbstverständlich* (self-evident or obvious), and only in difficult and problematic situations does the question of whether or not the act is legitimate arise. For instance, speech is determined by grammatical rules, but it is quite routine. Only when speaking an unfamiliar language it is necessary to think, to argue and to legitimate.

For Kohlberg, the form and structure of moral reasoning in problematic situations reveals the "moral grammar" which a person enacts in moral action. This may be true to a certain extent, but it does not take into account differences in moral grammars and the different stages in the development of moral grammars. Every act is moral. Acts should therefore be the empirical basis when analyzing moral reasoning, as opposed to the hypothetical discussion and consideration of acts. Kohlberg's theory is based on moral reasoning and not on moral action. Moral reasoning and moral action are only loosely connected, and because most actions are routinized, the actors are unaware of the decisions they are making when they are acting. Thus moral behaviour is based on moral grammar. In practical terms, to analyze human behaviour, it is better perhaps not to differentiate between motivational, cognitive and moral acts, since the subjects themselves do not do so.

In research, 50 scientists (25 natural scientists and 25 social scientists) were interviewed about the relationship between science and ethics, their aims, differences and the possibilities for change. The interviews were scored on the following scales:

1. which moral stage according to Kohlberg's theory they were in;
2. which degree of alienation they had;
3. the different disciplines were scored on a standardization scale.

Alienation was taken to mean "the control of human products over people". Human products which control people may be rules, beliefs, norms or material products such as streets and houses. They control us only when we believe that we cannot change them. Standardization was defined as the degree to which the behaviour of researchers and teachers in the discipline can be predicted by the material and the knowledge of the material which they use. Hence natural sciences are more standardized than social sciences. It was found that the higher the standardization of the discipline the lower the moral stage of the scientists, and the lower the moral stage the higher the alienation.

Further, the cognitive development of the discipline (its standardization) is connected with low stages of moral reasoning and perhaps also with a low stage of moral development and a high degree of alienation. For instance, many of the natural scientists also believe that there are two moralities, one for their discipline and one for everyday life. Most of them did not see that their scientific behaviour is ruled by norms, or that methodology is a rule system. They did not see that experimenting, for example, is prescribed by moral rules such as being exact, honest and hard-working.

In the high standardized disciplines scientists were more alienated, that is to say they were totally convinced that they did not have the possibility to decide what to do. They believed that they could not behave other than to conform to reality. They did not see that reality is made by human beings or that their behaviour is governed by rules made by human persons. It follows logically that they believe that they are not responsible.

There is a strong connection between how a person conceives and categorizes the world and the moral outcome of that person's behaviour.

In recent years I have done research into the socialization of scientists. For that research I needed a concept that was adequate for describing the effects of socialization. The concept had to fulfil two requirements:

1. it had to describe, better than concepts like "attitude", "value-orientation" and "personality trait" the complexity of dispositions which are integrated into a whole and nevertheless dynamic in structure;
2. it had to cover the two aspects of socialization: socialization as the reproduction of the structures of society, and socialization as individual growth and personalization.

The concept that did meet those requirements best was the concept of "habitus" (Bourdieu). *Habitus* is "a system of schemes of perception, thinking, judgment and action" which informs "within a given society the actions of the class members in very different aspects of life and work". *Habitus* is conceived as a "generative grammar for action patterns".[2] This grammar can be differentiated, and also different personal styles can be found, although there is an underlying structural unity. Hence every action has a collective and an individual aspect. This is why *habitus* as a model of an action grammar is useful as a concept for socialization effects. Linguistic grammars are learned by speaking, action grammars by acting. The development of the *habitus* is not something that only happens inside the individual when he/she is acting, the *habitus* is formed and supported also by selection processes (formalized and non-formalized), which influence status, situation and the make-up of the selected and the eliminated persons. One effect of these processes is the *habitus* of the academics, which can be found even in critical academics, who criticize the academic order or other academics. This *habitus* is the *habitus* of Gouldner's "new class". Gouldner reminds us that the "code of critical discourse" based on the idea of rational argumentation, helps to legitimize the privileges of the "new class".[3] A further effect of these processes is a special *habitus* for each academic discipline and profession.

Different situations were created to explore the different *habitus*, which could also be explored by the subjects themselves. The aim was to show that by becoming aware of a specific *habitus* it could be changed. A simple example is the view held by many scientists that science is an orderly collection of many truths and that it is learned from a "fundamentally" true basis. The theory of *habitus* can be applied to more serious issues. One obvious case is the fact that although many scientists are working on the production of materials of mass destruction potential, it is difficult to believe that any of them is interested in the destruction of planet Earth. By becoming aware of *habitus*-bound behaviour, and this is the main point of this paper, it is reasonable to suggest that it is possible to change the *habitus* to a more positive and useful concept.

---

2. P. Bourdieu, *Outline of a Theory of Practice* (transl. from the French), London, Sage, 1977; P. Bourdieu, and J.C. Passeron, *Reproduction in Education, Society and Culture* (trans. from the French), Cambridge, Cambridge University Press, 1977.
3. A.W. Gouldner, *The Dialectic of Ideology and Technology: the Origins, Grammar and Future of Ideology*, London, Macmillan, 1976.

Therefore in education, as Kohlberg's work in "The Cambridge Cluster School Experiment"[4] shows, it is necessary that each person is given responsibility in a just and fair environment, and that through discussion of cognitive moral conflicts and the practical continuation of this environment, the person can be led to a higher stage of moral development.

4. L. Kohlberg, E. Wasserstrom, and N. Richardson, "The Just Community School. The Theory and the Cambridge Cluster School Experiment", in *Collected Papers on Moral Development and Moral Education*, Vol. II, L. Kohlberg (hectographed manuscript) 1975.

REASONING IN SCIENCE AND ETHICS

GERRIT MANENSCHIJN

Many people, including the majority of scientists, do not anticipate any scientific problems with regard to the relationship between science and ethics. Scientific knowledge is objective and scientific judgments can be tested by observation of facts and by logical analysis. Hence you can only have two types of scientifically justified assumptions: empirical hypotheses and analytical propositions (logic and mathematics). If scientific propositions have been proved to be true, they will be generally accepted by everyone who is free, impartial and clear-headed. If some are not convinced, you can try to convince them by pointing out the predictability of scientific propositions: given a body in a certain system—for instance a planet in a solar system—and given also certain data about the mass, direction and speed of that body, we can predict with close accuracy just what the body will do when a certain force is applied to it. If the prediction comes true, then there is clear evidence of the truth of the hypothesis.

So much for the popular opinion of some scientists, which involves a positive view of science and technology. (Of course the terms "positive" and "negative" are used here in a scientific meaning, not in a moral one.) The other side of the coin is a very negative view of ethics. Moral judgments are utterances of private preference and subjective choice. They give a certain piece of information, but only about the pro and con attitudes of the persons involved. There is one simple reason for this: moral judgments cannot be empirically tested.

The consequences of this vision are disastrous for ethics. No scientifically accepted method exists to decide between alternative moral standards. Moral judgments are always subjective and private. There may occasionally be an agreement about moral standards, but that is purely accidental. Besides, such an agreement is extremely exceptional in modern society. A situation of moral disagreement is normal. In short: in the case of scientific judgments you can attain to cognitive certainty and factual agreement, whereas in the case of moral judgments such a possibility is principally and practically unattainable.

Is this opinion justified? I shall argue that it is too rigid an opinion, and founded on a misunderstanding of the essence of both scientific and moral reasoning.

Alasdair MacIntyre has pointed out that "the most striking feature of contemporary moral utterance is that so much of it is used to express disagreements; and that the most striking feature of the debates in which these disagreements are expressed is their interminable character ... There seems to be no rational way of securing moral agreement in our culture."[1] He gives three examples, the first is that of international security, the second of abortion and the third of justice. In international security policy there is a fundamental disagreement between (nuclear) pacifism on the one hand and a strategy of nuclear deterrence on the other. With regard to abortion there is a disagreement between the view that abortion is murder and the view that a pregnant woman has an indispensable right over her body, and that therefore she has a right to make her own decision on whether she will have an abortion or not. The third example shows the unsolvable problem of equality and freedom: equality demands that every citizen has equal access to health care and education, whereas freedom requires that physicians and teachers are free to practise on their own terms.

The problem is not that such moral dilemmas exist, but that there seems to be no rational procedure to decide which choice is best: for or against pacifism, for or against abortion, for or against equal opportunity.

Two presuppositions have been taken for granted: the first is that the contents of the judgments are left out of consideration; the second supposition is that the terms "positive" and "negative" have a scientific and not a moral meaning. But if we consider the contents of the scientific and moral judgments and if we make our judgments not from a scientific but from a moral point of view, then the perspective becomes quite different: science and technology are now accused of creating more social and moral problems than they have solved. The invention of nuclear fission has brought nuclear bombs and a permanent threat of destroying civilization on a worldwide scale, whereas the promising future of the peaceful application of nuclear technology seems to fade more and more. The car has brought almost as many traffic problems as it has solved, and the side effects of many medicines seem to be as harmful as their main effects are beneficial.[2] Humankind is on the threshold of a new cultural era: not a post-industrial world, but a post-personal world.[3]

How do we judge this dark picture of the impact of science and technology on our world? In my opinion it would be unreasonable to say that science and

1. *After Virtue, a Study in Moral Theory*, Notre Dame, 1981, p. 6.
2. Kurt Baier, "Technology and the Sanctity of Life", in K.E. Goodpaster & K.M. Sayre, *Ethics and Problems of the 21st Century*, Notre Dame/London, 1979, pp. 160–74.
3. Manfred Stanley, *The Technological Conscience, Survival and Dignity in an Age of Expertise,* Chicago/London, 1978, p. 11.

technology have caused all the social and moral problems we have to deal with. Science and technology do not exist independently, they are part of our culture. You cannot isolate them from the context of our culture and society. In our culture science and technology are supposed to make human life more comfortable. Modern medical technology has saved a lot of people from pain and death, scientific agriculture has made it possible to solve the problem of starvation (world hunger is no longer a technological problem, but a political and economic one); a car can give us a sense of freedom and the possibility of extensive travel, while modern education and information can put an end to illiteracy.

But we have overlooked two consequences. The first is that of undesirable side-effects. Medical technology has created victims of our medical knowledge and skill—the incurables whose dying process can be prolonged, but not prevented. It has solved many problems, but created new ones. That is the first forgotten consequence.

The second one is that the appearance of increased scientific knowledge and technological skill is deceptive. Baier argues: "It is not so much that there is a scarcity of the things wanted as that one person's doing what is necessary to satisfy his desires interferes with another's doing it also."[4] It would be very nice to go by car from Amsterdam to the beach in Zandvoort on a sunny day, if only few would do so. But sunny days are so rare in Holland that everybody will do the same thing resulting in enormous traffic jams and a lot of annoyance. Such a situation is not caused by science and technology, but by the selfishness of human beings. The real problem here is the insatiability of human desires, as Plato made clear. It is socially and practically impossible to adapt the satisfaction of your desires to the possibilities of technology, you must adapt the possibilities of technology to the satisfaction of basic human needs of all people all over the world. It is morally unacceptable that some part of the world population is starving and another abounds in food and other pleasures. But that is not a problem of technology but of social preferences.

A pragmatic view of verification and reasoning

It is important to realize that well-known positions in moral philosophy and moral theology are deeply influenced by contemporary positivist views of science.[5] In this context I stress the claim of logical positivism that moral judgments cannot be shown to be true or false, either analytically or empirically. In this view, only one thing concerning moral judgments could be said with certainty: they are partly expressions of feelings, partly commands.[6]

---

4. *Op. cit.*, p. 161.
5. Hermann Lübbe, *Sind Normen methodisch begründbar? Rekonstruktion der Antwort Max Webers,* in Willi Oelmüller, Hrsg., *Transzendental-philosophische Normenbegründungen,* Paderborn, 1978, pp. 38–49.
6. A.J. Ayer, *Language, Truth and Logic,* Harmondsworth, 1974, p. 7. See also W.D. Hudson, *Modern Moral Philosophy,* London, 1970, pp. 32–44.

Consequently the position of moral philosophy and moral theology was rather unsatisfactory, for nobody knew a satisfactory answer to this vehement attack. Some tried to defend an objective moral order, which was thought to be independent of the physical world, and could be known by revelation or intuition. One form of the first position is known as the divine command theory or theological voluntarism[7]—that the standard of right and wrong is the will of God; another holds that human beings cannot know what is right or wrong unless God reveals the moral law to us. The divine command theory broke down at the classical Judaic-Christian belief that God commands us to do what God wants because it is right and that God, being morally perfect, deserves our obedience,[8] whereas the theory of *Offenbarungspositivismus* fell short in explaining the human experience of a universal knowledge of fundamental moral rules and principles.

The second defence of objective moral order, existing independent of the physical world (intuitionism), was taken by Moore and others.[9] It had a lot of plausibility, for it seemed unquestionable that killing is intrinsically wrong and doing good to others intrinsically right. Nevertheless it was not ultimately a convincing theory. Both revelationism and intuitionism failed to show that ethics can refer to an objective moral order, independent of the physical world.

A third answer to positivism in science and non-cognitivism in ethics is given with the theory of act-deontology, also known under the inappropriate name of situation ethics. It accepts that ethics cannot be objective, claiming that it is the very nature of ethics not to be objective. It makes a virtue of necessity. In ethics all depends on moral choice. Not the contents of those choices, but the choices themselves are the essence of morality. The Christian variant of this theory claimed that it is the right choice that matters, and that the only standard of a right choice is the principle of "love" (*agapè*), but even this mitigated form of act-deontology was insufficient for two reasons: first, *agapè* is a principle that cannot be deduced from the choice itself, and second, *agapè* is too vague and general a principle to serve as a concrete action guide.[10] So situation ethics did not provide us with an appropriate alternative for non-cognitivism in ethics. We seemed to be in a deadlock.

Happily, it only seemed so. In reality the situation was less hopeless. First of all, it was pointed out that logical positivism was too rigid in holding that the

7. C.F. Henry, *Christian Personal Ethics*, Grand Rapids, 1957.
8. Victor Grassian, *Moral Reasoning, Ethical Theory and Some Contemporary Moral Problems*, Englewood Cliffs, New Jersey, 1981, pp. 25–27. Cf. H.M. Kuitert, "De Wil van God doen", in *Ad Interim, Opstellen over Eschatologie, Apocalyptiek en Ethiek, aangeboden aan Prof. Dr R. Schippers*, Kampen, 1975, pp. 180–95.
9. W.K. Frankena, *Ethics*, Englewood Cliffs, New Jersey, 1973, pp. 102–5 (Intuitionism), pp. 97–102 (Definitionism), and pp. 23–25 (Act-Deontology).
10. Joseph Fletcher, *Situation Ethics*, London, 1970, pp. 69–86. Cf. J.P. Wogaman, *A Christian Method of Moral Judgment*, London, 1976, pp. 14–32.

meaning of moral judgments can only be emotive,[11] whereas Popper and others proved that the verification principle itself was not wholly tenable.[12] Not deduction, but induction is the core of empirical investigation, because induction does not harmonize with verification, but with falsification. As is widely known David Hume was the first philosopher who convincingly argued for the principle of induction.[13] Space does not permit further exploration, but I agree with Derksen that falsification presupposes a moderate inductionism,[14] and in "normal science" (i.e. the way it is done in a scientific community) is rather exceptional.[15] As Derksen concluded: the purpose of science is twofold, first, instrumental success (problem-solving, improving the conditions of life), and, second, intersubjective knowledge of reality.[16] There must be a good reason for both purposes, theoretically as well as practically. Rationality in science is primarily connected with good reasons, rather than with irrefutable knowledge.

This illustrates an important trend in modern philosophy: the rehabilitation of practical reasoning as a rational way of deciding what to do. It is arbitrary to restrict rationality to methods of how to know, and not to extend it to reasons for what to do.

I conclude that there are grounds to defend a viewpoint both in science and ethics that people will have reason to do what they do or to believe what they believe. From this pragmatic point of view, taken by Toulmin and others,[17] it is reasonable to argue that there is much more resemblance between scientific and moral reasoning than is popularly believed. To summarize Toulmin's views in this respect:

—Conceptions about the natural world must be realistic and workable both theoretically and practically (this concerns both science and ethics).
—If and only if these conceptions are articulately expressed and open to public criticism, they can appropriately be classed as scientific. Since openness to criticism is a moral requirement as well as a methodological one, the moral dimension of public criticism is part of the question from the start.
—Reasoning in the natural sciences aims at a consensus, which was previously supposed to be the hallmark of (unscientific) moral deliberation.

---

11. Frankena, *op. cit.*, p. 105.
12. Karl Popper, *The Logic of Scientific Discovery*, London, 1959, passim. A.A. Derksen, *Rationaliteit en Wetenschap*, Assen, 1980, pp. 82–180. A popular introduction to Popper is Bryan Magee, *Popper*, London, 1973.
13. On Hume's induction problem there is a great deal of literature. A short and clearly written introduction is presented by A.J. Ayer, *Hume*, Oxford, 1980.
14. Derksen, *op. cit.*, passim.
15. Thomas S. Kuhn, *The Structure of Scientific Revolutions*, 1970. Cf. I. Lakatos & A. Musgrave, *Criticism and the Growth of Knowledge*, Cambridge, 1972.
16. Derksen, *op. cit.*, p. 303.
17. Stephen Toulmin, Richard Rieke, Allan Janik, *An Introduction to Reasoning*, New York/London, 1979, pp. 229–34.

—The professional institutions of science are organized to promote communal, collective goals. In other words: choosing subjects for scientific research is not so much a question of scientific preference as of social choice. But to get the best social choice you need a concept of a good and just society and standards of fair decision-procedures. That ultimately requires moral criteria.

However there are also differences between scientific and moral reasoning. In scientific reasoning one explains how things can happen; in moral reasoning one justifies why one is obliged to do what is to be done. In short, both in science and ethics argumentation is a technique for providing reasons for accepting a claim to truth or rightness. But science resorts to explanatory and ethics to justificatory reasons.

Toulmin's structure of argument

Stephen Toulmin and others have developed a useful model of argument.[18] It neither vindicates nor undermines scientific or moral procedures of argumentation, but rather suggests areas of genuine common ground. The structure and terminology are fairly technical and complex, but once mastered provide a valuable yardstick against which both scientific and moral rationality can be measured and compared. And our purpose in presenting Toulmin's model (with a few minor adaptations) is to identify similarities and differences between scientific and moral methods of argumentation.

Toulmin's structure of argument is shown in Figure I,* and an explanation of nomenclature follows.

EXPLANATORY REMARKS
—*Claim*: A demand for something which can reasonably be accepted as true, or as being one's legal or moral due. Instances of the first form are claims for factual evidence, causal relations or probable consequences (scientific reasoning), and of the second, claims for an action being one's duty, legal or moral (legal and moral reasoning).
—*Ground*: The underlying foundation for the claim to be accepted as solid and reliable. These may be generally accepted relevant facts (scientific reasoning) or valid descriptions of human conduct (legal and moral reasoning).
—*Warrant*: Justification of grounds by indicating what general rules, laws and principles make facts and descriptions relevant to the claim. Warrants may take the forms of laws of nature, engineering formulae, etc. (scientific reasoning) or of legal and moral principles (legal and moral reasoning).
—*Backing*: Generalizations, making explicit the body of experience relied

---

18. Toulmin, *op. cit.*, p. 78.
* Figures I to III are partially adapted from S. Toulmin, R. Rieke and A. Janik, *An Introduction to Reasoning*, London, Macmillan, 1979.

FIGURE I

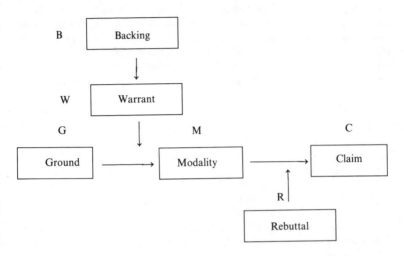

upon to establish the trustworthiness of the argument. In a scientific context backing involves pointing at currently accepted theories, which rest on adequate experimental evidence. In a moral context backing involves pointing at a basic moral rule that underlies the ethical warrant. Moral backing can go further backwards to pre-moral preferences; for example the preference that everybody is better off in a world of truth-telling than in a world of lying. This pre-moral stage of backing moral warrants indicates that moral basic rules and principles, though always resulting from a choice, are not arbitrary.

— *Modality*: The degree of certainty in grounding the claims. "Modal qualifiers" indicate this degree of certainty, which degree can be of almost 100% reliability, but often of only a certain percentage of certainty. In that case qualifications are used as "usually", "possibly", "presumably", "under the condition that" etc.

— *Rebuttal*: Production of evidence to refute a claim or the grounding of a claim. Unless we are faced by one of those rare situations in which the central step from grounds to claim is presented as "certain" or "necessary", we shall also need to know under what circumstances the present argument might let us down. Rebuttals may be foreseen or not, which means that any argument must be open to rebuttal. The rebuttal may be logical and factual evidence (scientific reasoning) or be another and over-ruling moral principle (moral reasoning). In practice a moral argument is always open to rebuttal, a scientific one not always.

Summarizing the Toulminian structure of argument: "The claims involved in real-life arguments are well-founded only if sufficient grounds of an appropriate and relevant kind can be offered in their support. These grounds must be connected to the claims by reliable, applicable *warrants*, which are capable in turn of being justified by appeal to sufficient *backing* of the relevant kind. And the entire structure of argument put together out of these elements must be capable of being recognized as having this or that kind and degree of certainty or probability and as being dependent for its reliability on the absence of certain particular extra-ordinary, exceptional, or otherwise re-butting circumstances."[19]

Attention must be paid to the following conditions of this structure of argument:

1. Arguments are meant to achieve one or another goal of a kind that involves changing other people's minds, not by using persuasive or commanding language, but by making appeal to the hearer's understanding. We produce reasons in order to convince him or her. We are open to objections and must perhaps modify or qualify our original assertion.
2. Argumentation presupposes the principle of reciprocity: others are equals and may have their reasons. Being open to argument means taking into account the reasons of other people.
3. Argumentation presupposes the rationality of moral discourses in making collective decisions in which rationality involves offering intersubjective valid reasons and an attitude of openness to argument.
4. The essential locus of reasoning is a public, intersubjective and social enterprise. Rationality is a necessary condition of public reasoning, not a sufficient one. A sufficient condition is the voluntary approval of the claim by recognizing the grounding as being appropriate.
5. Another necessary condition of reasoning is the sincerity and reliability of the participants in the discourses.
6. Reasoning is not a way of arriving at ideas, but rather a way of testing ideas critically. The task of reasoning in each situation is to enable the questioner to make the best decision about a particular issue, in particular circum-stances, within a particular forum and enterprise. ("Making the best decision" means that moral principles are always involved, since terms like "good" and "best" always have a moral connotation.)
7. The need for argument comes into play only if there is a conflict in answering questions like "how do you know?" and "what shall we do?" Argumentation always has to do with the practical goal of producing reasons at the right time for the right people in situations of conflict.
8. The forum of argumentation is in principle the public, but in reality there are many "forums of argumentation", such as:

---

19. *Ibid.*, p. 27.

—law courts (legal reasoning);
—scientific communities (scientific reasoning);
—medical specialists (scientific, legal and moral reasoning).

It is a characteristic of moral reasoning that the forum is always public, since it is a necessary condition of morality to choose as an autonomous person the action you think you are committed to. I call this necessary condition the principle of autonomy. This principle implies that a moral philosopher cannot be seen as an expert in making decisions in place of others. This indicates an essential difference from, for instance, an expert in engineering who is allowed to make decisions in engineering problems. A moral philosopher is never in such a position. It would be a violation of the principle of autonomy to make moral decisions in someone else's stead.

The resemblances and the differences can be demonstrated by comparing Figure II (scientific reasoning) with Figure III (moral reasoning). The resemblance is the same structure of argument, the same aim at a consensus or rational agreement between the parties concerned. The differences are at least threefold:

1. in scientific reasoning the argument concerns explanatory reasons, in moral reasoning justifying reasons;

FIGURE II: SCIENTIFIC REASONING

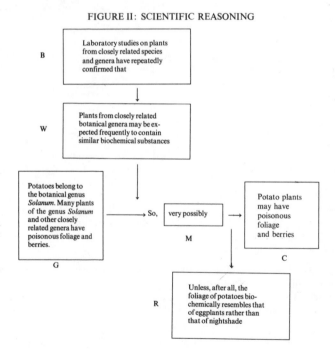

FIGURE III: MORAL REASONING

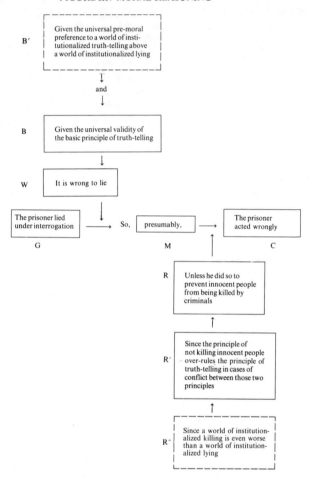

2. in scientific reasoning, if you can stay within the limits of the same theory, a contradiction between the pro-evidence (the backing) and the con-evidence (the rebuttal) says that at least one of them cannot be true, whereas a contradiction between pro-evidence (backing) and con-evidence (rebuttal) in moral reasoning does not say that, but obliges you to choose which of the two principles involved over-rules the other;

3. in scientific reasoning you normally stay within the limits of backing and rebuttal (if you cannot give a satisfactory explanation in that way you switch over to an alternative theory), whereas in moral reasoning you always can go beyond the basic principles of backing and rebuttal into the

domain of the pre-moral preferences for a certain concept of human wellbeing.

In the next example (Figure III) the domains signed through B' and R" indicate going beyond the limits of the moral argument into the domain of pre-moral preferences for a certain concept of human wellbeing. This going-beyond is necessary to point out the non-arbitrariness of the moral basic rules. It can be demonstrated that choosing these basic rules is a rational act of a rational person.

Now there are two questions to be answered. The first one is what are the basic principles used in a moral argument and how are they mutually related? The second is how is scientific reasoning related to moral reasoning in those cases (as is normal) in which scientific and moral arguments are both in question? These questions will be considered in the next two sections.

Basic moral rules and principles: how they function in moral discourse

In common with Beauchamp and Childress[20] I hold that there are three basic principles in moral argument:

1. the principle of autonomy;
2. the principle of non-maleficence and beneficence, in which the principle of non-maleficence takes precedence over the principle of beneficence when they come into conflict;
3. the principle of justice.

These principles do not have the same status. The principle of autonomy, defined as "the right to be respected as an autonomous agent and the duty to respect the autonomy of others in determining courses of action", can be considered as a necessary condition of acting as a moral agent. It is not a material moral principle, since the life-plan and the actions, chosen by the agent, may be judged as immoral and wrong. The moral value of autonomy has been a topic for discussion in Christian ethics, but I leave this question as it is. I agree with Immanuel Kant who said that an agent is autonomous if and only if he has a will to do good, and with John Stuart Mill who said that this will must be recognizable in the actions of the agent in question.

The practical consequences are significant: individual persons who claim the right to be autonomous are by claiming this obliged to act morally (according to their own moral criteria), and to respect equally the autonomy of others. In society as a whole social and political control over individual actions is legitimate only if necessary to prevent harm to other individuals affected by those actions. Last but not least the principle of autonomy says that in deciding what shall be the common good and what policies shall be chosen to promote

---

20. Tom L. Beauchamp, James F. Childress, *Principles of Biomedical Ethics*, New York/Oxford, 1979.

the common good, everybody shall count for one vote and every vote for one value. This is a form of democracy.

The role of autonomy in moral argument is that of a necessary condition of moral action. Autonomy implies that in all cases in which the common good is at issue the decision as to what to do has to be taken via democratic decision procedures and not by "experts", however skilled or informed they may be.

There is no fundamental difference between beneficence and non-maleficence. Beneficence refers to acts involving prevention of harm, removal of harmful conditions and promoting good (I agree with Frankena's precedential arrangement[21]). With regard to the role of the principle of non-maleficence in moral reasoning it can be said that the ultimate justification of questionable actions takes place with reference to this principle. Non-maleficence functions in the backing and/or the rebuttal of the argument. In Figure III, for instance, non-maleficence functions in estimating the precedence of R' (not killing innocent people) over B (truth-telling), since killing innocent people can be seen as a greater harm than lying to prevent that killing.[22]

The principle of justice is recognized to be a basic principle in any society, whatever the contents may be. I have analyzed the concept elsewhere, both the role and the contents of the principle of justice, and concluded that there are at least three criteria of distributive justice: everyone must be treated in accordance with his right, his merit and his need.[23] Suffice to say that it belongs to any concept of justice that if there exists an accepted arrangement of justice in a given society this arrangement should be applied impartially and equally to every member of that society. In moral reasoning justice functions as a standard of fair distribution of rights and duties, profits and costs, and assets and liabilities over all the members of the society.

The fundamental sense of justice is equality. If equal sharing is not possible, unequal distribution has to be justified by a standard of fairness. John Rawls has developed a theory of "fair unequality", but space does not permit me to expose his notion of fairness. I must refer to his famous *Theory of Justice* and to the summary of his theory in my book.[24]

The basic principles of morality are present in any society in an institutionalized form only. Musschenga, who made a profound study of the necessity and possibility of morality, made clear that you can never find the basic principles in a pure form, but always in the form of institutionalized basic rules. He pointed out that the principle of non-maleficence takes the form

---

21. *Op. cit.*, p. 47. Cf. Beauchamp, Childress, *op. cit.*, pp. 97–98.
22. Beauchamp, Childress, *op. cit.*, pp. 102–105.
23. G. Manenschijn, *Eigenbelang en christelijke ethiek, Rechtvaardigheid in een door belangen bepaalde samenleving*, Baarn, pp. 108–41.
24. Cambridge, Mass., Harvard University Press, 1971.

of at least three moral basic rules: not killing, not stealing, not lying. The ethnical, cultural and social context stipulates what count as acts of killing, stealing and lying. Conversely, it is possible to demonstrate that behind every institutionalized moral basic rule a basic principle is present as a final criterion of the rightness of the basic rules.

Musschenga argued that the function of morality is to promote acceptable forms of cooperation. In human society cooperation takes place via institutions. The institutional order of human societies, however, is an uncertain form of regulation. Institutional arrangements can, under the influence of unequal power and self-interest, be abused. It is the function of morality to be a counterpoise to tendencies of self-interest and abuse. Musschenga contends that morality is necessarily present in every society, and that it has a universal core of contents. That core consists of a certain number of basic rules (the prohibition of killing, lying and stealing) and two basic principles of legitimation (equality and reciprocity).

I want to take a step further and connect the three basic rules of Musschenga with the basic principle of non-maleficence and his basic principle of legitimation, reversely, with basic rules of institutional justice. I agree with Beauchamp and Childress that every rule presupposes a basic principle.[25] Consequently we must distinguish rules from principles.

Rules are rules of groups; they function as social action guides. Rules may be customary rules, describing how people behave, or rules of the game. They may be prescriptive rules, prescribing how people ought to act in social relations. Moral rules are always prescriptive, which means that obeying them or disobeying them depends on the acceptance of them by the people involved. In other words: the existence of a certain rule is dependent on the existence of a certain sort of critical attitude of the agents, an attitude expressed in principles.[26]

According to Richards the main difference between rules and principles is that principles do not depend on their literal and factual acceptance. "A certain principle (e.g. a principle of justice) could be accepted by no one at a certain period in history, and yet it may be true to say that what they are doing is wrong."[27]

The functions of principles in moral argument are as follows:

1. principles provide a final justification in a chain of standards; they are the final court of appeal of critical judgment of a reasonable and moral person;
2. an essential feature of a principle of action (e.g. a moral principle) is its generality: the lack of proper names; this indicates the general validity of moral principles: they are meant for everybody;

---

25. *Op. cit.*, p. 5; A.W. Musschenga, *Noodzakelijkheid en mogelijkheid van moraal*, Assen, 1980, pp. 159–218.
26. David Richards, *A Theory of Reasons for Action*, Oxford, 1971, pp. 13–14.
27. *Ibid.*, p. 14.

3. a crucial characteristic of moral principles of action is their universality: they apply or can apply to the actions of all persons, by virtue of their having the capacity to understand and act on them.[28] Hence principles are generally and universally formulated.[29]

Figure IV shows the structure of moral argument indicating the role and place of basic rules and principles.

According to Musschenga the possibility of a rational justification of morality is limited. Though it is true that every rational agent must come to the conclusion that morality is necessary—otherwise the war of all against all would be inevitable—it does not follow that the conclusion for any rational agent must be that he himself has to behave morally.[30] That is only true from a

FIGURE IV: THE STRUCTURE OF MORAL ARGUMENT

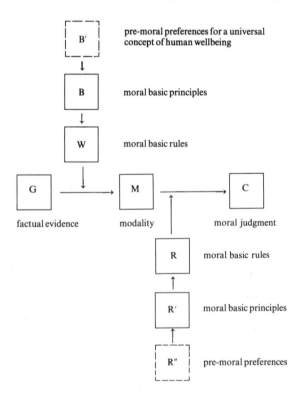

28. *Ibid.*, pp. 24–26.
29. R.M. Hare, *Freedom and Reason*, Oxford, 1972, pp. 38–40.
30. Musschenga, *op. cit.*, p. 268.

moral point of view. From an egoistic point of view it is rational to conclude that morality is necessary to prevent the war of all against all, but also, for yourself, that it is rational to be egoistic if all other people are moral. It is a matter of fact that an egoistic life-style is most successful if others are altruistic. Hence the line of the argument must not be that it is irrational to be egoistic, but unreasonable. To demonstrate this the procedure of universalization can be helpful.

It is a property of moral principles to be universalizable according to the formula: "If R counts as a reason in favour of a person A's doing X in situation S, then R also counts as a reason for a similar person to perform a similar act in similar circumstances." It is obvious that the problem will be how to determine if persons, acts and circumstances are similar. Since in all three cases similarity can never be 100%, we have to determine what is relevantly similar. To do that, we make use of the procedure of universalization. According to J.L. Mackie, there are three stages of universalization.[31] In the first stage, we want to rule out an irrelevant, mere numerical difference, namely the difference between one individual and another. What is wrong for one cannot be right for another merely because the two are not the same persons. There must be a morally relevant, qualitative difference. For instance: the differences between male and female are relevant for giving birth to children, not for being fully-fledged members of the church.

The second stage of universalization is the test of reciprocity: putting oneself in the other person's place. Imagine yourself in the other person's place and ask whether you can then accept it as a directive guiding the behaviour of others towards you. For instance: having a large income and an iron constitution it is easy to judge that everyone should pay in full for any medical attention required; but imagine that you are on a modest wage and have a child in bad health: do you still endorse the proposed rule? This stage of universalization rules out, among other things, cultural and religious prejudices against women.

In this second stage one imagines oneself in the other person's place, but still with one's own present tastes, preferences, ideals and values. Hence we are in need of a third stage: taking into account different tastes and rival ideas. That means that we are trying to look at things both from our own and from the other person's point of view at the same time, and to discover action-guiding principles which are acceptable from both points of view. In this stage an equal account of all actual interests is at issue. Since the principle of autonomy says that everybody has the right to determine his or her interests, it follows that if people can raise their voices and are able to vote, they have the right to do so. Hence apartheid will not come through the test of universalization. If people are not able to raise their voices, as in the case of unborn future generations, we are obliged to imagine seriously what their interests could be and what kind of world they would prefer to live in.

---

31. *Ethics, Inventing Right and Wrong*, Harmondsworth, 1977, pp. 83–102.

This third stage makes great demands on our own willingness to accept the values of others; we must go beyond psychological and private moral boundaries and that is not usual, especially for people with strong moral convictions!

Universalization does not factually eliminate egoism and egotism. It is a reasonable mode of argumentation, an attempt to convince, not to compel. The strength of moral reasoning is its reasonableness, not its violent power. If people refuse to be reasonable, any argument fails, both in ethics and in science.

Reasons for action—explanatory and justificatory

How do we relate explanatory and justificatory reasons for action?

My starting point is a truism: science is not an activity apart from humankind, but a specific human action. Human action can be called rational if and only if reasons can be given for acting in a certain way. Not only explanatory reasons, but also justificatory reasons. Now I would defend a position, taken by D.A.J. Richards, [32] that explanatory reasons are dependent on justificatory ones, and that therefore scientific activity is rational if and only if the goals of science can be justified by moral basic principles. The crucial point in this is Wittgenstein's thesis that understanding behaviour presupposes understanding the action guiding rules that are followed by the agent. Only rule-guided behaviour shows regularity, and regularity is a necessary condition of predictability. According to Richards the following scheme is representative:

1. A was in situation B;
2. A was a rational agent in that situation;
3. in a situation of type B, any rational agent will do X;
4. therefore A did X. [33]

From this abstract scheme one can see that the notion of explanatory reasons is conceptually dependent on the justificatory reasons, for I cannot, for instance, explain the behaviour of a chess-player unless I understand the rules of the game. The crucial difference between explanations in terms of reasons and in terms of mental causes is that the latter do not imply anything about the agent's rationality, whereas the former do. For instance: in terms of mental causes the actions of a madman can be explained as well as those of a rational man, but in terms of reasons for actions the madman's behaviour cannot be judged as rational or irrational. This crucial aspect must be left out of consideration. The madman acts, that is all that can be said. To judge human actions as being rational or irrational you need conclusive justificatory (or justifying) reasons.

---

32. *Op. cit.*, pp. 49–62.
33. *Ibid.*, p. 56.

The next step to be taken is the recognition that justifying reasons can be egoistic or moral. That was the topic of the last section. It follows from the argument as developed in that section that scientific activity is in need of justification with the help of the basic principles of autonomy, non-maleficence and justice. Given the generally accepted goal of science: promoting human welfare (or prohibiting human disaster), it would be illogical to determine science as a rational activity without taking into account the moral justification of the goals of scientific research.

Figure V suggests a possible way of interpreting scientific research in terms of explanatory and justificatory reasons.[34]

Whose concern it is to judge which reasons count as valid? First of all: it is the scientists'. Clearly the principle of autonomy holds with regard to scientists. They must act as autonomous agents, fully aware of their moral responsibility for what they are doing. Responsibility presupposes freedom to decide for yourself. We must be careful that science is not seen as an aid to the ideology of a leading group or even of the state as a whole. That would be disastrous for science as well as for society.

It follows that science must within set limits be free, especially in the domain of the scientific cycle. If a scientist has adequate, justifying reasons for doing his work there is no reason why others should interfere with what is not their business. Especially governments!

The scientist is held to be responsible, as is everybody in a democracy. On the other hand, however, it follows from the last section that a scientist should not justify his or her work with reasons of private morality, but with universaliz-

FIGURE V

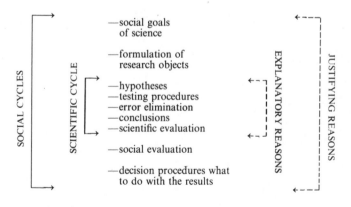

---

34. Cf. Henk Verhoog, "Filosofie en Wetenschapsbeoefening", in *Filosofie en Praktijk*, 2, 1981, pp. 121–131.

able basic principles of social morality. In so far as scientists are not trained in moral reasoning—and most are not—they should acquaint themselves with this important aspect of rational justification of human action. In my opinion moral philosophy and argumentation theories should be an essential part of scientific education.

In the domain of the social cycle, however, scientists have no more right than others to decide what the social goals of science will be or what to do with the results of scientific research.

COLLECTIVE SOCIAL DECISION-MAKING: IMPLICATIONS FOR TEACHING SCIENCE

GLEN S. AIKENHEAD

At the first International Symposium on World Trends in Science Education, Fletcher Watson argued that decision-making must play a major part in any science curriculum.[1] The wise use of knowledge enables students to assume the social responsibilities of attentive citizens or key decision-makers. Their country's survival and economic growth will depend upon the decision-making abilities of their society. Economic and social growth are also enhanced by innovations in science and technology. However, science and technology can create ethical conundrums and social problems which can only be resolved by collective decision-making; nuclear energy, over-population, warfare, energy shortage and medical advances are examples. This collective decision-making on social issues brings with it a host of variables inextricably inter-related, not the least of which are political, economic, ethical, scientific and ideological values: veritable sanctuaries for complexity!

Drawing upon theoretical perspectives, commentaries and experiences with collective decision-making, this paper has two main purposes: (1) to *clarify* what it means to make an informed decision on a societal issue related to science and technology; and (2) to *explore* some practical implications for teaching science at the secondary school level. Thus this paper is meant to explicate the consequences of Fletcher Watson's call for the inclusion of social decision-making in science curricula.

At first glance, teaching collective decision-making in the social context of science may look like political sensitivity immersed in a conceptual melange of interdisciplinary relationships and conflicting values. Appearances, however, are deceptive.

Clarity comes by unravelling several factors. Such factors include the interplay between collective and personal levels of decision-making; the psychological state of the decision-makers; the identification of different domains of society each with its own knowledge system and decision-making

---

1. "Science Education for Survival", in C.P. McFadden ed., *World Trends in Science Education*, Halifax, Canada, Atlantic Institute of Education, 1980.

tradition; the political interplay between the economic-social élites and counter-élites (including the professional conduct of scientists and engineers); and the distinction between constitutive values and contextual values.

The fact that technical information itself carries political-ideological baggage gives us reason to question the "objectivity" of science.[2,3,4] The ethical and political neutrality of the scientific enterprise is considered by many to be a myth. Public inquiries often uncover political, ethical or ideological biases among scientific and technical experts. Because political, ethical and ideological values influence professional judgment, there would appear to be some kind of communion between science and values. The nature of this communion deserves further attention in order to provide a clear and realistic perspective on thoughtful decision-making on social issues related to science and technology.

Values inherent in science and technology

Science has its own set of values which, like a constitution, guide scientists when they decide between, for example, competing theories or experimental methodologies. Such values and normative constraints are learned by the apprentice scientist and become an important aspect to his or her disciplinary matrix. Longino[5] refers to this set of discipline-centred values as *constitutive values*. By contrast, she points to the social context in which science and technology are done and refers to the set of ethical, ideological and cultural values as *contextual values*.

Those who believe in the neutrality of science contend that science is free of contextual values, not constitutive values. However, the value-neutrality-of-science position concedes that contextual values affect scientific and technological enterprises by influencing (1) the fields of research to be funded, (2) the explicit policy decisions over the technological implementation of science (debates over nuclear energy, for example), and (3) research methodologies which may conflict with ethical values. Longino concludes that contextual values do in fact seep into a scientist's set of constitutive values. Science is not value-free; it is value-laden with contextual values.

Using "value" in the sense of "contextual values", Graham[6] constructs a conceptual spectrum with "value-laden" at one end and "value-free" at the

2. D.E. Chubin, "Values, Controversy and the Sociology of Science", *Bulletin of Science, Technology and Society*, 1 (5), 1981, pp. 427–436.
3. P.J. Gaskell, "Science, Technology and Society: Issues for Science Teachers", *Studies in Science Education*, 9, 1982, pp. 33–46.
4. J.R. Ravetz, *Scientific Knowledge and its Social Problems*, New York, Oxford University Press, 1971.
5. H. Longino, "Beyond 'Bad Science': Skeptical Reflections on the Value-Freedom of Scientific Inquiry", *Science, Technology and Human Values*, 8 (1), 1983, pp. 7–17.
6. L.R. Graham, *Between Science and Values*, New York, Columbia University Press, 1981.

other end. He asserts that different scientific activities can be thought to lie on different parts of the spectrum. In cases where scientific and technological knowledge tends to be vague or inconclusive, science and technology are more vulnerable to contextual pressures and therefore they lie towards the value-laden end of the spectrum. Therefore ambiguity or inconclusiveness in technical information affects the decision-making by decreasing the importance attached to that information. But this shift in importance to a lowered status is not always recognized or acknowledged by experts. This causes the unconscious and/or explicit infiltration of economic, political, social and ethical values into scientific judgments. One case in point is the current acid-rain controversy between Canada and the United States, where a politically minded government agency rewrote the US scientists' report, causing it to conflict with the contrary findings of Canadian scientists on the detrimental consequences of acid-rain.

Scientific "objectivity" is one of several constitutive values communicated to students in science textbooks. However, science textbooks themselves have been shown to camouflage more subtle value-laden messages; for example, the idea that solutions to societal problems (such as acid-rain) only require more scientific knowledge and more innovative technologies—the "scientific-technological fix".[7]

When we investigate the constitutive values within science, we discover differences between the constitutive values espoused by the scientific enterprise and the constitutive values actually practised by individual scientists. For instance, scientists publicly revere objectivity but rely on subjective hunches in the privacy of their laboratories. Holton[8] reports that the value *suspension of belief* has a real and valid counter-value *suspension of disbelief* (tenaciously sticking to one's idea in spite of contradictory evidence), a value without which science could not progress. Holton explains this apparent conflict in values by distinguishing between two types of scientific activity, "public science" and "private science". Public scientific activity is reported in journals, conference proceedings and textbooks, while private scientific activity is carried out in laboratories and recorded in personal notebooks and letters. Scientific activity therefore embraces two legitimate, dialectical sets of values. Gauld[9] explores the implications of this conclusion for education by questioning the propriety of exclusively teaching the public-science set of values. These values by themselves propagate myths about the scientific enterprise; myths which erode thoughtful decision-making.

But how adequate are science's constitutive values for guiding research and

7. L. Factor & R. Kooser, *Value Presuppositions in Science Textbooks*, Galesburg. Illinois, Knox College, 1981.

8. G. Holton, *The Scientific Imagination: Case Studies*, Cambridge, Cambridge University Press, 1978.

9. C. Gauld, "The Scientific Attitude and Science Education: a Critical Reappraisal", *Science Education*, 66 (1), 1982, pp. 109–121.

development in the social context of the twentieth century? Some values appear anachronistic. Historical analysis draws attention to how modern scientific values were developed and shaped by seventeenth-century western European society. After reviewing the atomic bomb case study, Mendelsohn[10] concludes that some basic scientific values are simply inadequate. In their place he suggests four values that would help science interact congenially with its social context:

1. *Modesty*: the arrogance of contemporary science must be replaced by modesty... We must moderate our aims, and recognize that choices are made, and then make explicit the way in which we decide what we're going to do. The necessity of conscious choice makes us face directly the social elements involved.

2. *Accessibility*: science must be accessible to the general public in terms of understanding the enterprise (demystifying its knowledge), participating in important decisions (directions that research should take), and entering its professional ranks.

3. *Consideration of non-violent, non-coercive and non-manipulative research*: an oath similar to the Hippocratic oath of physicians would transform the relationship between science and society.

4. *Harmony with nature*: concern with the long-term effects of tampering with nature: will the activities we undertake benefit the quality of human life?

When we make a decision on a social issue, we must remember that knowledge and testimonies from science and technology will most likely become imbued with both constitutive and contextual values. Science and technology cannot be assumed to be as value-free as some science educators would have us believe.

Collective decision-making

GLOBAL LEVEL

Collective decision-making initiatives are reviewed and critiqued by Casper,[11] Krimsky[12] and Nelkin,[13] all of whom conclude that imaginative

---

10. E. Mendelsohn, "Values and Science: a Critical Reassessment", *The Science Teacher*, 43(1), 1976, pp. 20–23.

11. B.M. Casper, "Public Policy Decision-Making and Science Literacy", in D. Wolfle *et al.*, eds., *Public Policy Decision-Making and Scientific Literacy: Information Needs for Science and Technology*, Washington, DC, National Science Foundation, Report NSF–80–21–A6, 1980.

12. S. Krimsky, "Public Participation in the Formation of Science and Technology Policy", in D. Wolfle *et al.*, eds., *Public Policy Decision-Making and Scientific Literacy: Information Needs for Science and Technology*, Washington, DC, National Science Foundation, Report NSF–80–21–A6, 1980.

13. D. Nelkin, "Science and Technology Policy and the Democratic Process", *Studies in Science Education*, 9, 1982, pp. 47–64.

initiatives have suffered from (1) a lack of manpower and expertise to assess sufficient relevant data for the non-specialist; (2) a naïve view that scientific or technological facts are value-free and can objectively and deductively lead to a decision; (3) a lack of sufficient political-economic power and technical expertise necessary to ensure a balanced view among various adversaries; (4) an insincere concern for the public good, especially for those who will live on a day-to-day basis with the outcome of the decision; (5) an insulation from public view of the key decisions within government, the military and industry—decisions that commit large amounts of capital to a technological innovation, thereby creating a technology momentum, and only then offering public participation in *regulatory* decisions; (6) a stultifyingly narrow set of terms of reference for inquiries or study groups; (7) a conflict of interest in government, where agencies supporting the technological innovation are supposed to report "objectively" to the public; and (8) a termination of a forum or interchange when one side sees itself losing.

Action by an attentive public creates problems for administrative authorities by disrupting their efficient procedures and raising political dilemmas. Some critics have seriously questioned whether the public can adequately grasp the complexities and abstractions of the science and technology content to warrant the public's full participation. Research is needed to determine the extent to which a person's position on a social issue related to science or technology can be thoughtfully defended by political, social or ethical values without recourse to knowledge from science and technology. The success of the Cambridge Massachusetts Experimentation Review Board report, *Guidelines for the Use of Recombinant DNA Molecule Technology in the City of Cambridge* is often cited as an example of lay persons and scientists achieving a workable solution to collective decision-making on a societal issue.

Putting a collective decision into action involves political power and may cause ripples in the political-economic infrastructure within a country. Therefore before we can fully understand decision-making on a social issue related to science and technology we require at least an awareness of the issue's political-economic context and the associated power politics. Another question is what form of public participation in decision-making is favourable? Krimsky supports the use of a "citizen advisory board" which would have access to technical knowledge and scientific critics on all sides of an issue. Casper sees the greatest advantage in community action programmes funded without strings by governments.

STRATEGIC LEVEL
The complexity of collective decision-making may be simplified by considering some analytical strategies useful in making decisions on social issues.[14] For

14. G.S. Aikenhead, *Science in Social Issues: Implications for Teaching*, Ottawa, Science Council of Canada, 1980.

instance, a variety of social domains impinge upon collective decision-making. Thus one approach to decision-making is to decide which social domains are relevant. The next step in decision-making would be to identify the social domain in which the final decision will probably be made. Furthermore each aspect of society has its own knowledge base and its own tradition in decision-making. Thus the ways of making decisions differ significantly among lawyers, politicians, technologists and scientists. In other words the different social domains require different traditions for making decisions, contain different assumptions underlying each knowledge system, have different purposes in society, and in general view the world quite differently.

The credence of a scientist or engineer must change on shifting from a scientific or technical frame of reference in which he or she has some expertise, to a legal, ethical or political frame of reference. Scientific and technical information may be sought by social agencies. But its relevance will have to conform not necessarily to scientific constitutive values but to the norms of, for example, legal, ethical or political thought. Thus, scientific knowledge may, to the annoyance of some scientists, lose some of its distinctive character when used in another framework. This makes it susceptible to misuse or misinterpretation in other areas.

Since a thoughtful approach to resolving science-based social problems can begin by identifying various aspects of society germane to the problem, science students will have to learn a simple way of identifying these social groups; for example, by being taught to identify the principal aims of politics, art, logic, economics, technology, religious faith and science. Being able to identify simplified aims of various social groups allows students to analyze some "real life" situations. It also presents them with the perspective of examining science as *one* of several legitimate social enterprises.

When deliberating over a controversial decision, scientific and technical knowledge is more often used than ignored. Familiar examples include: using a political argument to evaluate scientific data in a court of law; using the biological concept of natural selection as a justification for a particular socio-political ideology ("survival of the fittest"); using Einstein's relativity theory as justification for accepting all viewpoints of ethics; and using the prestige of technology to justify dubious social, psychological and medical experiments. A thoughtful strategy for decision-making would be to avoid such abuses of science. Abuses may arise or go undetected due to a lack of understanding of the characteristics and limitations of science and technology.

PERSONAL LEVEL

Whenever a group collectively decides on science policy, on risks associated with technological advancements, or on the industrial production of technological innovations participants will have to make these same decisions individually.

15. I.L. Janis & L. Mann, *Decision-Making*, New York, Free Press, 1977.

Janis and Mann[15] developed a decision-making model based on conflict theory in counselling psychology. Counselling research places value on defensive avoidance behaviour (corporation executives and people who wish to quit smoking are popular subjects for this research). During counselling and training sessions people are required to fill out a "decision-maker's balance sheet". This process ensures that utilitarian gains and losses are considered for each alternative generated by the decision-maker, and that self-approval and approval from others are weighed explicitly. The assumption here is that each individual has the power to act on the basis of his or her decision. But for collective decision-making we do not necessarily live with the decision we advocate.

With this difference between personal/small group decision-making and with collective decision-making in mind, we shall tentatively apply the Janis and Mann theory to collective decision-making in the social context of science.

Wheeler and Janis[16] describe "the five stages of effective decision-making":

1. *Accepting the challenge*: If confronted with a challenge and if we perceive the threat or opportunity important enough, then we will make an effort to engage in the decision-making process. The motivation to do so relates to the degree of conflict we experience. The alternative to accepting the challenge is to exhibit defensive avoidance behaviour.

2. *Searching for alternatives*: Lists of viable alternatives are generated. The process includes a thorough consideration of goals and values relevant to the decision, and a careful vigilant search for a wide range of alternatives without eliminating any prematurely.

3. *Evaluating alternatives*: The advantages and disadvantages of each alternative are thoughtfully considered. The "balance sheet" serves to encourage a diligent search for reliable data relevant to the decision. Effective decision-makers will often reach a tentative decision based on the data gathered at this stage.

4. *Becoming committed*: A final decision is reached after reviewing the balance sheet. In addition strategies are formulated for implementing the decision. This includes contingency plans in case risks appear. Action is taken.

5. *Adhering to the decision*: Coping with set-backs is easier if decision-makers anticipate them and figure out counter-measures in advance.

These stages are validated by their apparent success in psychology counselling. However we need to select from the Janis and Mann model those ideas useful for clarifying collective decision-making. The extent to which we draw upon "the five stages of decision-making" is a measure of our focus on the individual involved in the process of decision-making. An effective decision-maker is one who shows vigilance in searching for information, carefully evaluating the

---

16. D. Wheeler & I.L. Janis, *A Practical Guide for Making Decisions*, New York, Free Press, 1980.

validity and reliability of that information and generally feeling committed to achieving a thoughtful decision. This effective coping pattern is called "vigilance". On the other hand "hypervigilance" is characterized by an indiscriminate openness to all information due to a tense conflict caused by a belief that a solution is possible but there is not enough time to search and deliberate. Alternatively in a "defensive avoidance" coping pattern, a person would treat information with evasion or selectivity (e.g. procrastinating, shifting responsibility or bolstering a pre-chosen position). A fourth coping pattern, "unconflicted adherence or change", follows the decision-maker's belief that no serious risk exists and thus one can afford to be indifferent to the decision whichever way it is made. Indifference, evasion, selectivity and indiscriminate searching are all information processing behaviours we wish students to avoid when they participate in vigilant collective decision-making.

Even for vigilant students who show discriminating behaviour and open-mindedness, the information they weigh may be unbalanced by its *vividness*. Vividness sways the decision-maker by the poignancy of the media bearing the message. Coloured photographs of aborted foetuses and the film "The China Syndrome" are examples of information vividness. Therefore the psychological state of the decision-maker will naturally lead to indifference, evasion, selectivity, indiscriminate or discriminate searching. Such states of mind will influence the tenor of collective decision-making on social issues related to science and technology.

SCIENTIFIC COMMUNITY LEVEL

Science teachers often assume that problem-solving skills developed in a classroom will transfer to decision-making abilities in real life. Savon[17] illustrates how the scientific community is ill-prepared to deal with "unethical" practices within its own ranks, especially when it affects financial support, research grants and industrial salaries. A professional career can be jeopardized if a scientist's or engineer's social conscience persuades him or her to speak against an industry or government. Stanley Adams was jailed in Switzerland for turning evidence over to the European Economic Community that led to the conviction of the powerful Hoffmann-La Roche pharmaceutical company. David Horrobin's research into possible medical risks of Hoffmann-La Roche's money-making "Valium" has been curtailed in Canada. Scientists were paid by Hoffmann-La Roche to criticize Horrobin's results and this affected his funding. Rosalie Bertell experienced repression from some of her colleagues because her results from low-level radiation research were bothersome to the nuclear power industry. Union Carbide scientists were hired to criticize her work publicly but anonymously. Her tyres were blown out on a busy highway after she had been warned by a nuclear power plant vice-president not to speak

---

17. B. Savon, *Science and Deception*, Toronto, Canadian Broadcasting Corporation, 1982.

about her research to a local medical school. Scientists and engineers themselves have participated on the side of industry and government in these defamatory activities. As Longino claims, contextual values *do* influence professional behaviour.

When it comes to collective decision-making on a controversial issue, the contributions from the scientific-technological community ought to be considered in the light of the fact that scientists or engineers can rarely escape the political context in which they do their research. Values, ideologies and reputations are all wrapped up in social issues related to science and technology—"political motivation hidden behind a smoke-screen of scientific confusion".[18]

Implications for teaching science

Collective decision-making on science-related social issues comprises one aspect of science-technology-society (STS) education. The STS curriculum movement has made some progress within post-secondary education. The idea of introducing it into secondary school science has encouraged people to wonder (1) if the cognitive complexity and "moral maturity" are too demanding for the average high school student; (2) what types of knowledge *of*, and *about*, science and technology are most useful; (3) what functional knowledge of society is required; and (4) how can science education institutions be reoriented to provide an interdisciplinary and socially contextual emphasis. In spite of the uncertainties that these questions raise, some science educators have piloted STS materials which involve students in making decisions on social issues.

CURRICULUM MATERIALS AND INSTRUCTION

Some projects have focused on the rationality of decision-making strategies. Other projects have dealt with collective decision-making in the STS context by means of simulations, projects and discussions. Simulations, for example, can define in concrete terms the inter-relationships among power politics, conflicting values, technical data and decision-making strategies. Four projects are mentioned for the implications they represent.

The Biological Sciences Curriculum Study (BSCS) pilot course, "Innovations: the Social Consequences of Science and Technology", explicitly teaches a decision-making model. This model is consistent with Janis and Mann's five-stage model, but does not include implementing action or adhering to the decision. On the other hand, *Science in a Social Content (SISCON) in Schools* invites students to contemplate how they might put their collective decisons into action.[19] The BSCS model emphasizes *values* as critical filters to the decision-making process. The importance of clarifying values is

18. A. Kantrowitz, *American Scientist*, 63, 1975, p. 509.
19. J. Solomon, *Science in a Social Context (SISCON) in Schools*, Oxford, Basil Blackwell, 1983.

stressed in the STS literature. The pioneering British project *Science in Society*[20] has received comments on "its 'establishment' stance and its failure to introduce for consideration radical alternatives and new frameworks for decision-making on STS issues". For example the essay "Science and Political Decisions" is perceived as concealing capitalist ideologies to the exclusion of social democratic ones. These comments are not repeated here as a critique of the project, but instead they serve as a warning that decision-making materials are vulnerable to ideological analysis.

At the risk of oversimplifying the intricacies of teaching collective decision-making in the social context of science, the following ten items are suggested as a guide to teachers who are considering decision-making instruction. While the guide emerges from our experiences in *Science: a Way of Knowing*,[21] it incorporates the essential ideas presented in this paper. To reach a collective decision on a science-technology based social issue:

1. *itemize* the domains of society which appear to be relevant to the issue;
2. *identify* which domain and/or agency is given the social authority, or has the political power, to make the ultimate decision (this process will probably require a class to sharpen the precise wording of the decision or series of decisions to be made);
3. *generate* plausible choices (beware of simplistic disjunctives!);
4. *predict* the short-term and long-term logical consequences of each alternative (including the social and psychological consequences);
5. *scrutinize* the data relied upon in making those predictions. What are the warrants and conditions for the knowledge claims made? To what degree are the data valid and reliable? Are any data presented in great vividness?;
6. *clarify* the values (constitutive and contextual) that seem to support or negate the various alternatives; also recognize the values inherent in the prediction of consequences;
7. *prioritize* the values (an individual task for students);
8. *weigh* the evidence, the probability of the various consequences, and the values underlying the alternatives;
9. *choose* one alternative, stating a thoughtful justification;
10. *clarify* the ways in which science and technology contributed to this choice (science and technology can contribute to the cause of the issue as well as its resolution).

These ten items do *not* constitute a linear logic. They delineate points that need consideration and reconsideration during the course of reaching a decision. This decision-making guide assumes that students are in a "vigilant" psychological

---

20. J. Lewis (project director), *Science in Society*, London, Heinemann Educational Books, 1981.
21. G.S. Aikenhead & R.W. Fleming, *Science: a Way of Knowing*, Saskatoon, Department of Curriculum Studies, University of Saskatchewan, 1975.

state of mind and will therefore actively choose an alternative instead of exhibiting indifference or defensive avoidance behaviour. It acknowledges the fact that a student's priority of values may change from one issue to another as a function of familiarity and emotional response to the issue.

Potential pitfalls

In a science classroom experienced teachers can discover unforeseen problems which may hinder decision-making instruction. Several important pitfalls are considered here.

LACK OF PREREQUISITE KNOWLEDGE

"Science: a Way of Knowing"[22] was originally intended to address the interactions between science and society. However, we shifted our goals when we discovered that students were unable to deal with the interactions between science, technology and society. The students had acquired such mythical views of science and were so ignorant of their society that they could not adequately discuss the interactions between the two. We altered our goals to address this critical deficiency in prerequisite understanding. Deliberation over societal issues related to science and technology will invariably be mediocre without a realistic appreciation of what can and cannot be done with scientific-technological methods and knowledge.

In order to make thoughtful decisions on issues associated with science and technology we need to be aware of the following:

1. the characteristics of science, including its aims, constitutive values (norms and counter-norms), human character (formally public and idiosyncratically private), socio-group dynamics, tactics for decision-making, methods for creating and extending knowledge, and its presuppositions and preconceptions;
2. the characteristics of technology, including its aims and values, how these change according to the context, its problem-solving techniques and design processes;
3. the limitations of scientific knowledge, scientific values, scientific tactics and scientific techniques, including the recognition that science is but one knowledge system among many, and an examination of the boundaries between science and politics, science and economics, science and religion, science and technology, and science and ethics; plus similar limitations in the realm of technology;
4. the interactions among science, technology and society, including the guidance of science via technological advancements, technology implementing scientific knowledge for the benefit of society, the ethical and ideological positions and political power inherent in such implementations, society's control over scientific and technological developments and the personal

---

22. G.S. Aikenhead, "Science: a Way of Knowing, *The Science Teacher*, 46 (6), 1979, pp. 23–25.

interpretations of one's community (e.g. as a consumer, voter or in relation to career planning).

CONSEQUENCES OF SCIENTIFIC CONTENT BACKGROUND

Teachers usually assume that a deeper understanding of scientific discipline-centred content leads directly to more thoughtful decisions on social issues related to science and technology, be it a national science policy or a local predicament. This is a pitfall and subject matter alone does not help. More importantly, decision-makers require:

1. the ability to apply broad scientific and technical principles and relationships (not memorized facts) that are pertinent to the issue in question;
2. an awareness of the characteristics and limitations of science and technology, and their interaction with society;
3. idiosyncratic information about the particular problem;
4. a way of dealing with the complexity of science, technology, politics, economics, ethics, ideologies, community preferences and values that bear on the decision;
5. explicit decision-making instruction, and practice in making independent, critical and thoughtful decisions which may conflict with the teacher's personal judgment.

There is another false assumption related to scientific content background: that a greater understanding of items 1 and 2 above will lead to greater agreement on the decision at hand. In fact ideological differences tend to be more poignant for scientists and engineers than they are for the general public. Therefore the goal of teaching decision-making skills for social issues is not to augment unanimity. Rather it is to encourage thoughtful decisions; decisions made while consciously aware of the guiding values and current knowledge relevant to the issue. Moreover, a teacher cannot expect unanimity or a "right" answer in decision-making lessons—this has important implications for examinations. But a teacher can reasonably expect most students to identify the roles that science, technology, values and ideologies play in the resolution of a societal issue.

NARROW RATIONALITY

Another potential pitfall concerns the difference between *rational* and *thoughtful* decisions. Those in society who consider themselves as watchdogs of rationality tend to have a narrow and absolute view of rationality. This narrow view feeds the assumption that the more scientifically-technologically literate people are, the greater their agreement on decisions related to science and technology. This ultra rationalist camp gives low priority to the values and ideologies that implicitly guide their rational decisions. Holton contends that the narrow view of rationality must be broadened if it is to be applied realistically to science. In order to extricate this paper from the quagmire of "rationality" the label "thoughtful decision" is used instead of "rational decision".

The distinction between thoughtful and rational decisions reaps benefits in the classroom where we find students repulsed by their perception of a mechanistic, logical positivist ethos inherent in scientific and technical thinking. They usually assume a holistic humanistic ethos in their thinking and tend to resist "rational" decisions. Hence a teacher has a better chance of engaging students in "thoughtful" decision-making as long as their holistic humanistic view of the world is accepted as thoughtful. Because holistic preconceptions will conflict with mechanistic preconceptions, decision-making will seldom be unanimous. More importantly, a teacher can fall into another pitfall by not acknowledging holistic humanism as being thoughtful!

LACK OF COMMUNITY ACCEPTANCE OF ALTERNATIVE IDEAS

A scientist's or engineer's economic-ideological persuasion often affects the expert testimony given in court or at inquiries. Given the controversies that exist among experts, a teacher must anticipate similar controversies among parents. Some communities are less tolerant of controversial issues than others. For instance in many American communities teachers perceive the questioning ethos of scientific inquiry as contrary to their community's values and norms. Consequently these teachers refrain from inquiry instruction. Teachers who successfully deal with controversy in their classroom judiciously involve parents in some manner, thus avoiding a political pitfall.

POLITICAL POWER

The last potential pitfall concerns power. If we develop students' ability to reach decisions on social issues related to science and technology, we are taking them to the door of political action. This may or may not be our intention. If it is not then the political power issue becomes a potential pitfall. One of the disadvantages ascribed to increasing public awareness of a science-related social issue is the fact that an attentive public often finds itself disenfranchized of the power to take action. When this happens a conflict arises between, for example, an industry—the economic-social élite—and a community—the counter-élite.[23] If by developing students' abilities to reach decisions on social issues we encourage political action and conflict, then this instruction may be threatening to those in the community who identify with the élite. Some science teachers find themselves in a community that generally accepts reasonable political action on the part of students. These teachers often use the political action as a methodology for teaching decision-making on societal issues.

Such are some of the pitfalls inherent in the clarification of informed scientific and technological decision-making and its practical implications for the teaching of science at secondary school level.

---

23. T. La Porte, *Provisional Model of Technology and Social Change*, Berkeley, University of California at Berkeley, Political Science 188, 1983 (mimeographed).

ETHICS IN THE CLASSROOM: GOALS AND EXPERIENCES

HARRIE EIJKELHOF

I was trained as a physicist. I have worked as a science teacher in Zambia and in the Netherlands, and I have been active in curriculum development during the last seven years. So I shall deal with ethics in science education from a rather pragmatic view. I will not discuss the various theories of moral development. I have been asked to pay attention to the way the political dimension of social questions could be presented in schools. I will first explain why it is necessary to include ethical issues in the science curriculum. Then I will discuss the aims which should be pursued in science education. This will be followed by six examples, selected from curriculum projects with which I am familiar.

Social change

The last forty years especially have seen the development of many new items in the fields of consumer products, transport, communication, health and defence. Some of these changes have had an enormous long-term impact: "New knowledge and new technological developments also alter the range of choices and alternatives open to people. Such choices often necessitate a reconsideration and restructuring of personal and social values. Unanticipated consequences of technological innovation can result in ethical questions."[1]

At the same time it is clear that society is becoming more pluralistic: individuals and groups have different perceptions about individual and societal wellbeing, different definitions of trade-offs, benefits and costs, and different images of the future. Even scientists and technologists are giving strongly conflicting advice on issues which are a matter of public debate.

As a third important change I refer to the general trend in many countries to involve more citizens in public decision-making. In many of the issues on

---

1. Mary C. McConnell, "Teaching about Science, Technology and Society at the Secondary School Level in the United States", *Studies in Science Education*, 9, 1982, p. 13.

which decisions are required, scientific and technological aspects are important.

How far are these social changes reflected in science education in schools? Does science education aim to prepare students to live in the society of today and tomorrow?

Science education at present

Science education at secondary school level is still based on the traditional idea that science is neutral, value-free and insulated from questions of value and ethics. In physics teaching efforts are mainly aimed at the principles of physics as such.

Applications only come in if they serve as tools for understanding the basic principles. Education is not aimed at the use of knowledge and skills in personal and social life. In many countries examinations dominate the teaching of science in upper secondary schools. In the words of a "converted" teacher: "Sociology and government were problems for other classes and for teachers who wanted to avoid the hard discipline of preparation by staging impromptu moral wrestling matches in their classrooms."[2] I believe that this describes the situation in most science classes all over the world. So, generally speaking, my answer is negative on the question about the role of science education in preparing students for real life.

Of course I know of exceptions, and later I shall mention some examples. Other hopeful signs can be found in several policy documents of science teachers' associations[3] and international bodies,[4] and proceedings of recent science education conferences[5].

Ethical goals in science education

In my view science education must be changed from "teaching scientific knowledge and skills" to "learning how to use scientific knowledge and skills in personal and social life". This includes learning how to deal with the new range of choices and alternatives open to people, how to cope with the pluralistic

2. Clifford Swartz, in his editorial "The Moral Equivalent of Physics", *The Physics Teacher*, 17, September 1979, p. 354.
3. Education through Science, Association for Science Education, Hatfield (UK), 1981. *Science-Technology-Society: Science Education for the 1980s*, NSTA Position Statement, NSTA, Washington, DC, 1982.
4. UNESCO Congress on Science and Technology Education and National Development-Paris 1981, Final Report, UNESCO, Paris, 1982. I also refer to the activities of the Committee on the Teaching of Science (CTS) of the International Council of Scientific Unions (ICSU), CTS-Newsletters, Malvern, UK.
5. Integrated Science Education Wordwide, Report of the ICASE–Conference, Nijmegen, 1978. *World Trends in Science Education*, proceedings ed. C.P. McFadden, Atlantic Institute of Education, Halifax, 1980. A second symposium was held in Nottingham, UK, in July 1982; the proceedings are in press (G.B. Harrison, ed.).

character of our society and how to participate in public decision-making.

For this purpose science education should make use of controversial issues in which knowledge and skills are used in the context of values held by individuals or groups. In real life opinions are often presented as facts and it is very difficult to detect this if one is not trained to do so. A systematic reflection on responsible decisions and actions would be very useful when dealing with controversial issues. And that is what I consider to be ethics.

The three main aims of ethics in science education should be:[6]

— *Recognizing ethical issues*: Students frequently think in terms of a single solution. The influences of family, churches and certain newspapers might have been important, but in general science education works in that direction: most exercises only have one correct solution. Students must learn to recognize that often several alternatives are possible and that the choice between these depends not only on facts but also on the opinions and beliefs of those involved. This of course also requires an acknowledgment of freedom of choice and some doubts in the dominating social consensus. This might have a liberating effect on students as does being aware of alternatives.

— *Developing analytical skills*: Being able to discuss value-issues rationally can be very helpful in deciding complicated issues or clarifying the opinions of oneself or other people. It provides students with the tools for a more articulate and consistent way of justifying their moral judgments and of describing the process of their ethical thinking. Developing analytical skills should be coupled with the development of communication skills such as listening and the ability to paraphrase others' points of view.

— *Tolerating and reducing disagreement*: Ethical issues often arouse very emotional reactions. These should not be avoided, but left to themselves they might block communication between people. Students should learn how to express their feelings and ideas on an issue, and accept other points of view. They should then proceed to seek out points of agreement to reduce conflict and feel able to disagree without fear of reproach.

Achievement strongly depends on the availability of curriculum materials, on the attitude and skills of the teacher, the receptivity and capabilities of the students and the general ethos of the schools. Kohlberg and his colleagues have spelled out several kinds of experience which can stimulate the active problem-solving efforts necessary for moral development:[7]

---

6. I have been inspired to write this paragraph after reading Daniel Callahan, "Goals in the Teaching of Ethics", in *Ethics Teaching in Higher Education*, D. Callahan & S. Bok, eds., New York, Plenum Press, 1980, pp. 61–74.
7. This part of Kohlberg's work is summarized by Thomas Lickona, "What Does Moral Psychology Have to Say to the Teacher of Ethics?", in *Ethics Teaching in Higher Education, op. cit.*, pp. 110, 111.

a) being in a situation where seeing things from other points of view is encouraged;
b) engaging in logical thinking, such as reasoned argument and consideration of alternatives;
c) exposure to moral controversy, to conflict in moral reasoning that challenges the structure of one's present stage of moral development; and
d) exposure to the reasoning of individuals whose thinking is one stage higher than one's own.

To offer these experiences to students requires changes both in the content and in the teaching methods in science education. You cannot teach ethics by simply lecturing about it!

This list of four experiences is not complete: Kohlberg mentions two others which relate to the general climate of the school. They are beyond the control of the science teacher but no less important:
e) having the responsibility to make moral decisions;
f) participating in creating and maintaining a just community whose members pursue common goals and resolve conflicts in accordance with the ideals of mutual respect and fairness.

All this sounds very nice in theory and has been well described in several publications. But what does it mean in practice? Is it at all possible to integrate ethics into science education? What consequences does it have for students, teachers, curriculum-developers, teacher trainers and others involved in education?

Some examples of ethics in science education

The examples I will present here are local and refer to work in physics curriculum development. This does not imply that developments in this field are not taking place in other places. In the FRG (Institüt für die Pädogogik Naturwissenschaften),[8] the United Kingdom (Science in Society,[9] SISCON-in-schools[10]) and the United States (Biological Science Curriculum Studies)[11,12] several projects introduce ethics into science education. They should be studied. The reason I have taken examples from the Dutch scene is

---

8. Examples of IPN-courses are:
   —Einheitenbank Biologie, Aulis Verlag Deubner, Köln, 1981.
   —Stoffe und Stoffumbildungen, Ernst Klett Verlag, Stuttgart, 1979.
   —Curriculum Physik für das 9. und 10. Schuljahr, Ernst Klett Verlag, Stuttgart, 1976.
9. *Science in Society*, teacher's guide and readers, J.L. Lewis, ed., London/Hatfield, Heinemann/ASE, 1981.
10. SISCON-in-schools, J. Solomon, Oxford/Hatfield, Basil Blackwell/ASE, 1983.
11. For recent information on BSCS see ref. 1, pp. 1–32.
12. One of the few teachers' guides on values in science education is: Charles R. Barman, John J. Rusch, Timothy M. Cooney, *Science and Societal Issues: a Guide for Science Teachers*, Cedar Falls, Iowa, Science Activity Fund/Price Laboratory School, 1979.

that I have been involved in it myself and so I am able to use information from the primary sources: curriculum-developers, evaluators and teachers.

"Physics in Society"[13] is an optional part of the national physics examination programme and originates from a book published by the Free University. The book deals with various controversial areas such as energy, noise, transport, nuclear arms and informations systems, and uses scientific arguments to indicate various areas of disagreement. Elsewhere it shows what kind of choices are available in developing countries with traditional, advanced or intermediate technology. The final chapter contains information about the development of the relation between science, technology and society. Five different views are presented on problems relating to the development of science and technology: the capitalist system is at fault, experts are at fault, developments cannot be held in check, science itself is at fault, mankind is at fault.

In many schools the book is mainly used as background reader while the main activity is writing an assignment on one specific point from the book, based on information from a variety of external sources which are consulted by students themselves. This option is very popular among pre-university students. Evaluation studies show that most topics from the book are found interesting and important by 80–100% of the students. A notable exception is the last chapter on the relation between science, technology and society which is of a more abstract character and is generally more difficult.

Evaluative studies showed that about one third of the teachers detected some fear among their students of being judged on the basis of their opinions. Some were also inclined to parody the views of their teacher. This might have to do with a feeling of insecurity among students who are not familiar with testing situations in science education in which more than one truth is possible. Moreover marks are terribly important to students in their examination year and some are prepared to go to great lengths to improve their marks. But most teachers found that these feelings of insecurity diminished after a class discussion on the criteria of judgment. After the examinations we have not heard any complaints from students about the fairness of marking—which does not necessarily mean they were all satisfied with their marks!

Since 1972 the Project Curriculum Development in Physics (PLON) project has been trying to develop a new physics curriculum for general secondary education.[14] The main aims of the project are the growth of students' independence and sense of social responsibility, and the practical usefulness of

---

13. H. Eijkelhof, E. Boeker, J. Raat, N. Wijnbeek, *Physics in Society*, Amsterdam, VU-Bookshop, 1981. For a description of the course and some results of evaluation studies see: H. Eijkelhof; J. Swager, *Physics in Society*, New Trends in Physics Teaching IV, UNESCO, Paris, 1983.
14. More information on the PLON-project and on PLON-materials is available from PLON, P.O. Box 80.008, 3508 TA Utrecht, The Netherlands.

physics teaching in real life situations. In the units physics is therefore linked with the actual environment of students and with specific developments in society. A lot of attention is paid to decision-making and moral issues in general. From the 35 units published so far I have made a selection.

Units 1, 2 and 3 are for use by students aged between 15 and 16. Units 4 and 5 are part of the curriculum of 17 to 18 year old students.

Unit 1: "Stop or keep moving"[15]

Six means of transport (walking, cycling, motorcycling, car, bus and train) are compared from the point of view of one of the following: energy consumption, use of materials, speed, traffic noise, space taken on roads, and traffic safety. Each group arranges the six methods of transport in preferential order, giving arguments for each choice made. Questions to be answered are: How did you compare them? How did you define your criteria? Why did you compare them as you did?

The results of all groups are presented in the form of a matrix. A class discussion then follows on one or more of the following:

a) Which points of comparison are most important?
b) Are there other points relevant to decisions about transportation which have not been investigated (price, comfort, air pollution, employment)?
c) Are these points equally important for short and long journeys?
d) Which is more important to you: personal comfort or the effects on society as a whole?
e) Who should take decisions about transport (e.g. government, car manufacturers, road builders)?
f) How essential is transport?

Some findings of evaluation studies on this unit are:

— Using a matrix is difficult for many students, it is much easier to evaluate means of transport on one point only.
— Strong teacher guidance is necessary at the following stages: introduction of the unit, control of the plans of investigation of all groups and the final class discussion.
— In the final class discussion students often show more intuitive confidence than with regard to the results of their own investigations.

Unit 2: "Water for Tanzania"[16]

The unit deals with the choice of a water pump to be used in a developing country. Students are "employed" by the so-called Technical Advisory

---

15. Koos Kortland, "Schüleraktivitäten im Physikunterricht—Entwicklungs-tendenzen in den Niederlanden", in *Zur Didaktik der Physik und Chemie*, Vorträge auf der Tagung für Didaktik der Physik und Chemie/Würzburg, September 1982, Kiel, GDCP, 1983, pp. 52–63.
16. An English translation will be published by NIB, Zeist, 1983.

Bureau for Africa (TABA) which has been asked for advice by the Ministry of Overseas Development about a pump to be used in a village in Tanzania to pump drinking water from a depth of five metres. The Ministry specifies six requirements with which the pump should ideally conform: cheap fuel, locally available materials, easy maintenance, cheapness, no water pollution and sufficient capacity. These requirements relate to the construction of the pump, its physical working principles and the living conditions in the village.

After familiarizing themselves with these conditions groups of students study practically four different pumps. They take an existing model to pieces or construct a model themselves (which takes much more time!). Each group demonstrates its pump to others and explains its working. They also give advice about their pump based on the six criteria, including other advantages and disadvantages which could influence the final decision. All pumps are then compared in a class discussion, and the class votes about the advice to be sent to the Ministry. The arguments which were found to be most important and the manner in which physical and technical knowledge influenced the discussions are noted.

The unit is very much appreciated by students, 86% of whom want it to be part of the physics curriculum.

Unit 3: "Nuclear weapons and/or security"

The central theme of this unit is the dilemma: "security through deterrence" versus "security through disarmament". It is introduced with two texts which advocate these two viewpoints. It is then explained that security has different meanings for different people depending on what they value to be important. The next section deals with three aspects of the role of physics and technology in the arms race and the proliferation of nuclear arms. In this way students get some idea of the interaction of physics, technology and society. Information is given on the effects of nuclear weapons and differences in comparison with conventional arms. In the final stage students make an inventory of possible actions to be taken by different people and their effectiveness.

Not all teachers working with PLON-materials are willing to include this unit in the physics curriculum. They give the following reasons:
— "Too much politics, not enough physics!"
— "I don't know the answers to these problems myself."
— "My personal involvement is so strong that I cannot participate objectively in class discussions."

At one school the unit was banned by the school board because it was considered non-physics and too biased. In my opinion the various opinions are presented in a balanced way.

Unit 4: "Ionizing radiation"

"How acceptable is the risk of ionizing radiation?" is the central question of this unit. To answer it the unit breaks it up in sub-questions such as: Who takes advantage? Who bears the risk? How large does one estimate the risk to be? How could the risk be reduced or avoided?

Three fields of application are selected: nuclear power, nuclear arms and health radiation. Before working in groups on one of these applications students are informed about the physical and biological effects of radiation. They must gather information from various external sources such as libraries, hospitals, power stations and civil defence institutes.

Unit 5: "Matter"

The central theme of this unit is the development of notions of matter from the time of the ancient Greeks up to the present. The final section deals with recent developments in elementary particle research. By means of texts, a card-sorting exercise and a video-tape students get an idea of what is going on in big centres of high energy physics research such as CERN, Fermi-Lab, Stanford and Brookhaven. At the end of the session students must formulate advice to the Dutch government on the continuation or withdrawal of its financial contribution to CERN (approximately 50 million guilders a year). The advice should not be merely yes or no but must be based on arguments.

This unit has been used at our experimental schools for the last two years. A few students were not satisfied with it. They told us: "We have been shown various theories of matter and one after the other they were found not to be fully satisfactory. Even quarks may not be the ultimate truth. We don't like this. Physics should tell us how nature is and not how nature might be."

In some classes students were at first quite opposed to a discussion on the financial contribution to CERN: this was not considered to be physics. After watching the video tape their opinions changed completely. After seeing pictures of the huge accelerators of CERN, Stanford and Fermilab, fierce arguing started spontaneously about these "fantastic" or "ridiculous" aids to this kind of research in physics. Arguments were raised about the cultural and scientific value of this kind of research, its spin-off, its high costs and its safety.

These five units are illustrative of the PLON project. Others, such as one dealing with energy, would also fit very well into this set.[17]

Some lessons learned

I have described some of our experiences with particular units. Now I would like to dwell on the more general experiences related to ethics in physics education. I have classified them into four categories: student activities, teacher training, opposition and choice in the curriculum.

---

17. I refer to two publications: J. Kortland, "Energy in the Future", in *Proceedings of the GIREP Conference 1981*, Nuclear Energy/Nuclear Power, ed. G. Marx, Budapest, 1981, pp. 361–364; Piet Lijnse, "Energy and Quality", paper to the conference "Entropy in the School", Balaton, May 1983.

It is not always easy to devise suitable student activities. Some topics, such as nuclear energy and nuclear arms, are not suitable for practicals! Others are not easy to handle within the constraints of the present educational system—large and lively classes and external pressure from examinations. Of course reading a text is relevant to most topics. But there is a danger that this kind of activity is all too often used. Many students do not like a lot of reading, are easily bored by texts or have difficulties with the reading level. Mary McConnell recently described reading level problems in the BSCS programme "Innovations: the Social Consequences of Science and Technology."[18] On the other hand reading cannot be avoided when dealing with rather complicated social, technical and physical issues. As a result of these experiences we have developed the habit of asking ourselves always: What do we expect the student to do in and outside the classroom? We must not only keep in mind what a student should learn but also how.

Teachers have a certain image of science and science education; it is deeply rooted and difficult to change. Their own education at school, university or teacher training college has a long-standing influence. Innovations in curricula require teacher training and guidance, which is not easily organized in times of enormous cuts in educational budgets and in a country in which teachers are already overloaded with extra duties and responsibilities. In the PLON-project we use regular teacher meetings in which experiences with previous units are evaluated and in which teachers are preparing themselves for new units. So meetings are of practical use to both teachers and curriculum developers. We also use detailed teachers' guides with lots of ideas, hints and other sorts of information for teachers to choose from. We suggest possibilities and offer supportive arguments; they choose.

Anyone who is trying to introduce controversial issues into science education must be prepared to face resistance from various quarters. We mentioned earlier some hesitations among teachers to deal with nuclear arms in physics classes: they felt too much involved with the issue, considered themselves not to be experts in this field—or else they defined physics in a more narrow sense. Official bodies are opposed to it because they want to avoid politics in science classes or are concerned about an increase in the general level of frustration among pupils about the future of society.

But not only teachers and official bodies have to be convinced of the importance of ethics in science education. Some students do not want to express intimate feelings and personal views in the presence of their classmates. Others already have a view of the identity of science which would make anything out-of-bounds which relates science to other realms of knowledge. At PLON-schools we faced problems with students from other schools which teach science in a more traditional way. Other students had chosen science as

---

18. See ref. 1., pp. 25, 26.

an examination subject so as to proceed with studies in tertiary education in which science is required. They feared that moral discourse would endanger their preparation for further studies.

We have the feeling that the reluctance of some students is partly caused by the fact that learning to deal with the applications of science is experienced as different from learning how to solve a pure-physics exercise. The students might feel that this latter activity is more tangible and therefore regard it as more instructive. Applications have to do with real life and are more complicated and difficult.

Curriculum developers have to face another problem.[19] Science curricula all over the world show signs of being overloaded. Adding new aims to science education—how to deal with moral issues, for example—could make matters worse. So choices have to be made; something familiar might have to be dropped. To propose this may not make you very popular because there are always teachers who happen to be fond of the topic you wanted to scrap. But it must be done: we are convinced that each new suggestion should be accompanied by one or more suggestions for something to be deleted. Discussions on this matter should not be held on the topics as such (nearly all topics might be taught in an interesting way) but they should be based on the *aims* of science education.

A second problem of choice appears when dealing with complicated issues (e.g. nuclear controversies, the consequences of micro-electronic innovations). These issues are so vast that they could each fill the time available for a full science curriculum! Many could well be part of other subject curricula. So certain examples must be carefully selected in such a way as to avoid presenting a too reduced and distorted picture of the issue on the one hand, or, on the other, diluting the curriculum so much that science as such virtually disappears.

The goals I began by setting out can only be attained subject to certain conditions. The first is the acceptance by all concerned that students are different: they have different interests, different backgrounds, different abilities, different styles of learning and different views. Without respecting these differences any progress towards the main aims of ethics in science education would be hopeless. In the past science education has paid too much attention to differences in cognitive abilities.

A second condition is the willingness of those in charge of science curricula to create possibilities for student activities which stimulate moral development. In most curricula little space is currently available. Thirdly, I wish to stress the readiness of teachers to accept that science education should make a contribution to the moral development of students. As a consequence they

19. H.F. van Aalst, H. Eijkelhof, "A Perspective on the Implementation of Science-Technology-Society-Education at Secondary School Level", *Proceedings of the Conference Risk and Participation*, Amsterdam, VU-Bookshop, 1983.

must be prepared to adapt some of the scientific content and methods of teaching.

The fourth condition concerns the educational climate in the schools. I think this climate is of utmost importance. I do not see how moral development can be promoted in a school in which students are not allowed to carry responsibilities, in which someone with a dissenting opinion or deviant behaviour becomes an outcaste and in which conflicts are not resolved in a respectful and fair way.

The moral development of students must be promoted as an integral part of science education.

IMPLEMENTING EDUCATIONAL INNOVATIONS

Alfred K.F. Schermer

The situations

It is generally agreed that there is an urgent need to pay more attention to the ethical implications of science in science education at all levels. But how are we going to introduce new ideas, new approaches, new strategies into our work and that of our colleagues? How do we implement new educational approaches?

There are roughly three situations in which you have to deal with adoption and implementation:

1. you wish to innovate your own teaching;
2. you wish to innovate the teaching of your colleagues in your own institution or school;
3. you wish to innovate teaching and education outside your own institute.

In the first situation—you wish to innovate your own teaching—all seems very simple: you simply do it! But as you know sometimes you intend to do things but you just don't take action. Intention is not the same as action. You may have adopted your own plan but there are things that hinder you from implementing it. I believe that the factors that hinder you are much the same as in the other two situations.

In the second situation—you want to improve the teaching inside your own institution—things are more difficult. To begin with, there are more persons with different characters to deal with. You are likely to be misunderstood and you do not have the same control over the actions of others as over your own. Your colleagues may adopt your proposal, but then either not implement it, or implement it in a way you had not intended.

In the third context—you want to innovate teaching outside your own system—things are still more difficult for the following reasons:

1. you have still less control over situations;
2. communication is more difficult because the people out there almost certainly speak a different language; and

3. you know less about the conditions and influences that act upon the teachers.

Here too your proposals may not be adopted, may be adopted but not implemented or may be adopted and implemented, but not implemented as intended!

Role of concerns

Why is it that people—including yourself—often readily adopt a new idea but have great difficulty in implementing it? This is because they have concerns! This seems to be a trivial statement but it isn't. The work of Fuller (on teacher training) and later of Hall, George, Rutherford and Loucks on implementation has shown the usefulness of this concept by recognizing what they call the various "stages of concern". Their research has indicated that a person who is confronted with an innovation goes through a fixed pattern of concerns. If one wants to persuade other people to implement an innovation it is essential to know their concerns. The concept of "stages of concern" also gives insight into what concerns they have already left behind and what concerns may come up next. The stages of concern are as follows:

awareness	(1)	A person in this stage is just aware of the innovation but has no great concern about it.
informational	(2)	The person is interested in the innovation and wants more information about it.
personal	(3)	The person is (well) informed about the innovation. He or she is uncertain if he can meet the requirements and is concerned about his role and the relationships in the new situation.
management	(4)	Attention is turned to processes and tasks the innovation will bring with it. Questions of time, resources and (classroom) management are in focus.
consequence	(5)	Not until now a genuine concern arises about the profits the innovation will bring for the pupils. What is the worth of the innovation if a teacher is able to carry it out properly (stage 3) and if the management of the innovation is no longer a problem (stage 4).
collaboration	(6)	Concern is now about cooperation with others in the use of the innovation.
refocusing	(7)	In the last stage the person begins to think about alternatives to do some parts of the innovation better than the original proposal. The person has a clear understanding of the pros and cons of the innovation (stage 5).

FIGURE I: CONCERNS PROFILE OF A TYPICAL NOVICE TO AN INNOVATION; HIGH SCORES ON INFORMATIONAL AND PERSONAL CATEGORIES

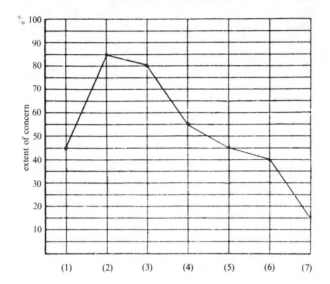

At the beginning of the implementation process one may expect that the concerns about information and particularly about the consequences for oneself are high. With the help of a questionnaire (the Stages of Concern (SoC) questionnaire), one can measure the extent of the concern. It is possible to draw from the scores on this questionnaire a profile of a person's concerns. Figure I shows a typical profile of a person in the beginning or just before an implementation process.

On the other hand one can expect quite a different profile from someone who has been using an innovation for some time. Figure II shows high scores on "consequences", "collaboration" and "refocusing".

Clearly it is useful if one wants to persuade one's colleagues or others to implement an innovation to know what concerns they have. If a person is largely concerned about the implications the innovation will have for him personally other arguments and other support must be used/given than when his concerns are about what his pupils actually learn from the innovation.

Perhaps these things are partly a matter of commonsense, but in my opinion the questionnaire is very helpful in digging up real concerns, even if a person has some theoretical knowledge. So, when you want to change your own teaching, the concept of the stages of concern and the questionnaire are helpful in analyzing your own concerns. Many people sometimes rationalize their

FIGURE II: CONCERNS PROFILE OF A TYPICAL EXPERIENCED USER OF AN INNOVATION; SCORES ARE HIGH ON CONSEQUENCES, COLLABORATION AND REFOCUSING CATEGORIES

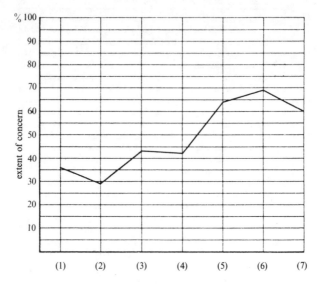

problems away by indicating the wrong causes; this process helps you to focus on the real ones.

The concerns of teachers regarding an innovation can be so great that they do not adopt it. But concerns need not to bear on an innovation as a whole but on particular elements. Fullan and Pomfret[1] have indicated five dimensions on which curriculum change can have an impact. A teacher can have distinctive concerns about each of these five dimensions:

1. subject matter or material;
2. organizational structure;
3. role/behaviour;
4. knowledge and understanding;
5. value internalization.

He can for, for instance, be concerned about materials at the level of "consequences for pupils" while he is concerned at the "personal" level about his role in guiding a discussion.

The extension of the concept of stages of concern with dimensions of the innovation is very fruitful in understanding the complexity of the process of innovation. In the case of introducing ethical issues into science education

1. M. Fullan and A. Pomfret, "Research on Curriculum and Instruction Implementation", *Review of Educational Research*, Vol. 47, 1977, pp. 335–97.

there is likely to be a change in every dimension. Very often there is a change in subject matter. For example in a unit on food in a biology/chemistry course, producer countries of fats and oils (most of them third world countries) and world market prices of those raw materials are mentioned in order to show that these prices are very low as compared with the price of butter in the European Economic Community. For a biology teacher who formerly only dealt with the digestion of fats under the influence of bile, or for the chemistry teacher who explained double bonds in fatty acids, these items are new!

Now discussions revolve around opinions, viewpoints, arguments, interpretations and so on. Many science teachers find it very difficult to guide such discussions: they have difficulty with their role, tending to steer the discussion into the clear waters of information-giving rather than through the unknown sea of argument. They also may have difficulty in organization if a project prescribes that students go out of the school to seek information on a social issue on their own, or if small groups are to work on parts of the project which must then be linked to the whole. Most teachers have very little knowledge of "ethics" and they do not see clearly what the objectives of this kind of teaching should be. They tend to shuffle those difficult subjects away to social studies, economics or religious education. They have not yet internalized the fact that it is very important to show all the relationships of a subject taught in science with other fields of knowledge and experience!

From adoption to implementation

We have seen that concerns about parts of a curriculum play an important role in adoption and implementation. We must now take a closer look at the relationship between adoption and implementation.

Until some ten years ago only the term "adoption" was used. It was an uncontested assumption that if a curriculum was adopted it was carried out as well. We now understand far better that adoption is only the first step, the first decision. Only then does a process of implementation start in which the innovation is more or less carried out. In the course of this process many decisions on parts of the innovation are to be taken, and at every decision point there is a chance that that particular part of the innovation will not be implemented or not implemented as intended. So in the case of a whole curriculum extending over a great number of periods, the probability that the whole curriculum will be implemented as intended is rather low.

How bad is it if a curriculum is not implemented as intended? That depends on the position the curriculum-makers take and hence on the design of the curriculum they make. There are two opposite positions curriculum-makers can take: they can be convinced that the users will implement the curriculum as intended. Then they will tend to prescribe in detail what the teacher has to do, what material he has to use, etc. They tend to take the place of the teacher to create the largest guarantee possible to achieve the objectives of the curriculum. They will think that essential characteristics of the innovation can be wrapped in appropriate learning materials. If this well prepared route is not followed many important objectives of the curriculum will not be achieved. This position is called the "fidelity approach" because users must follow the prescriptions faithfully.

If on the other hand curriculum developers think that users will automatically make changes, they will construct their curriculum in a different form, they will take much trouble to communicate the essentials of the curriculum to the users and they will offer alternative ways to achieve the objectives of the curriculum. Perhaps they will urge the users to develop alternatives more fitted to their own environment. This is called the "adaptive-approach".

It should have become clear that the most important part of a curriculum is the intended learning outcome, that is, what pupils are supposed to be able to do after instruction. It is about WHAT is to be taught not HOW. Some people say this *is* the curriculum. It can be left to teachers to plan ways of instruction to achieve these intended learning objectives.

Others are not so confident that teachers are able to do this on their own. They feel teachers need help. It is the extent to which this "help" is given that makes the difference. Nobody will say that a teacher or anybody else should be able to achieve a certain set of objectives with his (or her) pupils without using teaching and learning materials. It is the degree to which those materials are prescribed that makes the balance tip to the side of the fidelity approach or the adaptive approach. So some influence on how the teaching is to be done is included in this conception of the curriculum. *A curriculum is then defined as a set of intended learning outcomes plus a set of proposals on how they can be achieved.*

We have seen that personal concerns have considerable influence on the adoption and implementation of an innovation. An innovation can take the form of a large- or small-scale curriculum project presented to teachers. They may adopt it or not, implement it as intended or not. Such a curriculum impinges primarily on five dimensions. The introduction of ethical and social issues has implications for all five dimensions. It will be clear why until now the introduction of these issues in traditional science education has not been a success! We have seen that curriculum-makers can take two extreme positions, the fidelity position and the adaptive position. And we can now define a curriculum as a set of intended learning outcomes plus a set of proposals (including materials) on how to achieve those objectives.

Once a curriculum has been adopted, what are the factors which determine to what extent implementation will take place? Some have been mentioned already, but I will now deal with them systematically.

The following list is derived from the article by Fullan and Pomfret[2] on implementation research, that turned out to be a landmark in this field. I have added one factor to this list, "development", because the way a curriculum is

---

2. *Ibid.*

developed is vital. At present curricula are mostly developed part by part and tried on a small scale first, so "development" and the initial implementation overlap to a certain extent. The better these trials are the greater the guarantee that the curriculum will be adopted and implemented. Nowadays the adaptive approach gets the upper hand. Trials must be true field trials with true consumers. This means that one must be careful to extrapolate from trials with reliable and yet critical teachers and pupils.

In addition to "development", Fullan and Pomfret specify the following fourteen major factors which determine implementation:

Characteristics of the innovation
  0. Development
  1. Explicitness
  2. Complexity

Strategies
  3. In-service training
  4. Resource support
  5. Feedback mechanisms
  6. Participation

Characteristics of the adopting unit
  7. Adoption process
  8. Organizational climate
  9. Environmental support
  10. Demographic factors

Characteristics of socio-political system
  11. Design questions
  12. Incentive system
  13. Evaluation
  14. Political complexity

We shall consider them briefly in order:

Explicitness: One of the most important requirements of an innovative proposal is that it should be made very clear. However trivial this may sound, research has shown that teachers often have only a vague idea what the innovation is about, or what is the purpose of certain curriculum materials. I have already indicated this in the paragraph about the dimensions of curriculum change. This is mostly because curriculum planners seriously fail to communicate carefully the intentions of the project and their reasons for designing the curriculum in this way[3] to the teachers who are supposed to use it. The demand for explicitness calls for a teacher guide, which does not tell

---

3. D.F. Walker, "A Naturalistic Model for Curriculum Development", *School Review*, Vol. 80, 1971, pp. 51–65.

the teacher what to do, but explains to him why various activities are proposed.

Complexity: As we have seen, a curriculum change consists primarily of five dimensions all of which are influenced by ethical factors. So for many teachers this kind of innovation is complex and difficult to perform even if they feel it is valuable. Furthermore many teachers have little knowledge of ethics and philosophy, and therefore have doubts about the value of all their efforts. They must change their role from lecturer to discussion leader, and read up on new subject matter. Furthermore the classroom changes from an orderly lecture room into a market place where students engage in unstructured discussion.

Problems with changing roles are the most frequently reported difficulties teachers meet with in implementing innovations. Failure to innovate is mostly caused by failure of teachers to change their roles. That is not to blame the teachers. My point is that innovators vastly underestimate the complexity of change for teachers.

In-service training: Because implementation of an innovation is complex and difficult teachers should be given professional help. Few teachers are used to designing alternative learning activities intended to achieve the kind of objectives advocated here. They have depended on traditional subject matter and their own (also rather traditional) routines. So it is not enough to make a good (explicit) proposal; provision must be made for further support and training. In my experience role-playing is a very valuable teachnique for "unfreezing" teachers from their routines.

Resource support: Where necessary teachers must be supplied with resources and materials they don't have in their schools. Very often materials are new and specific for a certain innovation. It will greatly facilitate the implementation of an innovation if those materials are provided or can be borrowed.

Feedback: Feedback and participation are powerful instruments for facilitating implementation. Teachers have a great need to share and talk about their experiences. Nothing is more suited to enhance their commitment than a willing ear. Therefore developers must plan time to listen to teachers when the implementation process has started. They must also plan for interactive networks among teachers wherein they can exchange their experiences.

Participation: It is generally assumed that participation of teachers in development greatly enhances implementation. Research does not support this view: the evidence is inconclusive. But even if it made a difference it would hardly be practical because only a few teachers can participate in developing a project. Only in a very sophisticated project—with a large coordinating staff—real participation of all teachers becomes possible. Therefore it is much easier for the developer to participate in implementation. Developers should have at least some time for evaluative studies which can be used to do this. They must go into class-rooms, observe lessons and talk to pupils and teachers.

Most important of all they must carry out some of the learning activities they designed.

> If there is one finding that stands out in our review it is that effective implementation requires time, personal interaction and contacts, in-service training and other forms of people-based support. Research has shown time and again that there is no substitute for the primacy of personal contact among implementers and between implementers and planners.... All of this means that new approaches to educational change should include longer time perspectives, more small-scale intensive projects, more resources, time and mechanisms for contact among would-be implementers.[4]

Developers must not only develop a curriculum but must also develop extended support.

On the next group of factors, the characteristics of the implementing unit, I shall be brief. Some will be re-examined under the heading "incentive system" (fourth group).

A developer must be very sensitive to the *organizational climate* of the school where an implementing teacher works. This is only possible if the developer regularly visits schools. He can then influence the adoption process of the innovation he propagates. Thereby the factors mentioned play an important role. Teachers must be informed about in-service training, resources, feedback and participation. The building of an interactive network starts the moment innovative proposals are offered to a school. A new point here is the trend to address whole sections or departments of schools. Those sections form the natural interactive network for a teacher, and implementation seems to be more likely to occur if all the teachers of a section are equally well informed. In this way *environmental support* for the teachers can be increased. A developer cannot change the *demographic factors* of a school. But he can design alternative materials for certain school settings, or help teachers to develop those materials in the light of the intended learning outcomes, possibly adjusted to local contexts.

From the fourth group of factors, "characteristics of the socio-political system", I will deal more fully with the *incentive system* and make only short remarks on the other three. It is a *design question* how one can introduce ethical and social issues in education, secondary as well as tertiary, on a larger scale. What plans and strategies should be designed? It seems certain that there are no large funds available to start a major project. An alternative might be to start with small-scale projects with the facilities available in universities and teacher training colleges and to aim at a "snowball-effect". It is a question of

---

4. Fullan and Pomfret, *op. cit.*, p. 391.

policy why social and ethical issues penetrate so slowly into education by comparison with computers. It is a matter of *evaluation* at this level (evaluation of course being also an element within the curriculum) if introduction of social and political issues in science education makes any sense: are the intended learning outcomes achieved and do they function (later) in society?

These are questions on a macro-political level that deserve a separate elaboration. I have chosen to concentrate on the position of the educator, which is why I neglect other important aspects, except one: the incentive system.

Incentive system: The incentive system is a very important and much overlooked area in implementation. To put it plainly it is about what a teacher gets in return for his efforts in introducing something new into teaching. The personal cost for teachers, in terms of energy, time, and even trauma involved in learning new skills and roles (and unlearning old ones!) is often high. But by and large teachers are expected to bear those "costs" at their own personal expense! Complaints by teachers about lack of time, overloading and multiple demands are largely neglected. In some large-scale projects teachers receive facilities, but these are always less than the real time (and energy!) invested. Moreover those resources are drying up. So we will have to think carefully about other possible incentives.

Teachers have a great need for acknowledgment and affirmation. And innovators who come to tell them that they should do something new will very easily give the impression that they disdain the present teaching of the teacher. Therefore developers must first observe teachers and affirm the good things in their teaching. The build-up of an interactive network is of major importance because talking with other teachers about both innovation and about their "normal" teaching will give them part of the acknowledgment they need.

The "environmental support" for the teacher in his or her own school will be a major incentive. It makes a difference whether a teacher earns appreciation by his colleagues for his innovative efforts, or whether he encounters resistance and indifference. The developer must therefore look for possibilities to strengthen this kind of environmental support for the teacher. This may be done by talking to colleagues, heads of departments and school leaders, showing (and thus having!) not only interest in an innovation but in the school scene as a whole. It always amazes me with how little investment of time one can as a visiting observer gain "environmental support" for both the teacher and the innovation!

As you will have perceived I have gradually shifted into the language of secondary education and curriculum development, which is the domain which holds most of my interest. But I am certain that what I have said applies as much to university and college teaching and education of the general public.

In conclusion, adoption and implementation are quite different processes and people have different concerns for different dimensions of an innovation. Innovators can take a fidelity approach or an adaptive approach. It is my opinion that the adaptive approach offers greater chances for implementation. There are many important factors at various levels which hinder or promote implementation. In my opinion the presence or absence of explicitness, extended support and incentive mechanisms are the most important.

I will end with a quote by Williams:[5]

> Always think about implementation problems and always worry that others are not thinking about them, but do not expect major improvements to come quickly.

---

5. W. Williams, "Implementation, Analysis and Assessment", *Policy Analysis*, Vol. 1, No. 3, 1975, pp. 531–66.

SCIENCE EDUCATION
AND SOCIETY

SUMMARY OF THE DISCUSSION
Howard Davis

The group attempted to specify the general public's attitudes towards science. The core problem was diagnosed as the remoteness of the scientific community from everyday life and thought; its language, mode of reasoning and elitism. Among the general public (taken for the purposes of discussion to mean all non-scientists), responses to science range from blind faith to fear, scepticism or antipathy. Members of the group considered examples of these diverse attitudes and the potential for misunderstanding which exists where the conduct of science is detached from questions of value, ethics and religion. Many people have no grasp of scientific method. Their image of science is formed by the practical uses of the machines they work with and the goods they buy. The commercial motives behind a great deal of research and development are reflected in popular utilitarian views of applied science.

The questions raised in the opening discussion were taken a stage further by Charles Birch in an extended critique of what he called "the substantialist prejudice" in science or the view that the universe can be represented as a collection of independent entities (whether individual cells, small organisms or human beings) subject to external relations like the laws of mechanics. The method is reductionist: "We murder to dissect." Religion is simply irrelevant to this perspective. An alternative way to see nature, according to Birch, is to begin with what we understand of ourselves and our human dependency on relations which are internal, subjective and creative. The metaphor of God as the "Divine Carpenter" needs to be replaced by another more ecological model.

Many in the group responded sympathetically to Birch's critique.[1] It is easy

---

1. Elaborated in C. Birch and J. Cobb, *The Liberation of Life: From Cell to Community*, Cambridge University Press, 1981.

to recognize that the whole is more than the sum of its parts, whether the subject is the human personality, the family or the entire universe. However, there was debate in the group about the status of the proposed alternative model. Is it simply a competing scientific model or something more? How can it be tested? How does it relate to religious world-views? How can the mechanistic paradigm be transformed into an ecological one? It was noted that alternative approaches like F. Capra's have been gaining ground among scientists and that the fear of catastrophe is motivating a wider search for better integration between science and ethics. The same fear motivates questions being asked by the wider public.

The group spent much time considering some alternative proposals in greater detail. The general question was put: "Is there a methodology for a *holistic* science?" (The term "holistic" was used interchangeably with "ecological" to refer to scientific attempts to perceives the unity of the universe and life in all its manifestations). The examples discussed were alchemy, Goethean phenomenology, the ideas of Fritjof Capra, and the "Deep Ecology Movement". Most members of the group found something of interest in these different approaches, although some are generally too obscure, inaccessible and incomplete to be anything more than suggestive of what a transformed science might be like.

H. van Erkelens described how the western alchemical tradition which preceded the emergence of modern science emphasized the unity of nature, humanity and God. It contributed to important discoveries which have gone unrecognized in the history of science which looks backwards only from the contemporary western scientific standpoint. J. Bockemuhl, arguing for Goethean phenomenology as an alternative to Newtonian science, spoke of its applications in biodynamic farming. Some felt that it offers a viable and sustainable alternative to industrialized farming methods, but only on a small scale. There was scepticism about the general applicability of the approach in complex industrialized societies. Discussion of Capra's *The Tao of Physics* and *The Turning Point*, where an explicit link between modern physics and eastern mysticism is made, returned to the question of religious understanding in relation to scientific method. Piet Born wondered why there is little movement among Christians in the direction of a more holistic science. "Process" theologians and philosophers are moving in this direction, but they have only a small following.

The group reached no general conclusion about holistic alternatives to modern western science. It is clear that the "substantialist" view has taken a very firm hold of science and science education. But the examples discussed yielded several issues which need to be explored if there is to be a transformation of science for the future. First, the history of science must be revised to take into account certain undercurrents which have stressed the unity of nature and humanity. Second, the Christian understanding of creation and creativity must free itself from prevailing mechanistic interpretations.

Third, the churches must recognize and respond to new possibilities for convergence between science and religion.

It was agreed that the scientific search for order in the universe does not lead to any overall sense of meaning. While some scientists may be content with this, especially as the search for order and structure has been enormously successful, there is a deep desire to make some sense of things as a whole and to find a meaning which is both highly personal and at the same time all-embracing. Since science cannot provide this answer to the question of meaning, it was felt that scientists and teachers should shun "scientism" and be more open and flexible in their understanding of matter, life and the universe.

A lack of consensus about alternative "scientific" methodologies did not prevent the group from debating the values which should inform scientific practice. The chosen starting-point was Everett Mendelsohn's suggestion for the values of a new science: modesty, accessibility, non-manipulation, harmony with nature and equal involvement of men and women. But it was not clear how to put these values into practice.

The accessibility of science to the general public and participation by the public in important decisions were seen as priorities. The obstacles to these were acknowledged to be the sheer scale and complexity of modern technology and the decision-making process. If participation is to be the norm, there must be greater emphasis on small-scale person-orientated technology as well as good stewardship of the earth's resources. However, it was noted with regret that "hard" science attracts more funds for research than these "softer" approaches. E. Lindberg spoke of the economic context which works against alternative science and technology. The constraints do not arise from immutable economic "laws", he argued, but from the myths of economic "science" which serve to conceal the inherent inequalities of the market system. Economy dominates technology, so that things which cannot be produced "economically" are not produced at all. The transfer of inappropriate technologies to less developed countries illustrates the urgent need for open discussion of the assumptions behind theories of development. A further obstacle to participation was felt to be the idea of domination over nature, which may be partly attributable to a misunderstanding of Genesis.

The group was unanimous in the view that there are formidable obstacles to the transformation of science which cannot proceed without substantial changes in the structures of economics and society. But it was felt that the churches have a major role and responsibility to seek ways of communicating a new understanding of science and technology to scientific practitioners and to the general public. Participants were able to share their experiences of a variety of church-related programmes and other organizations or projects designed to further this process of communication and transformation, including several referred to already. None provides a definitive model for action but all contribute to the exploration of the ethical issues arising from contemporary science and technology.

REPORT

The present impact of science on society

There is much misunderstanding among the general public of what science is and what it holds for the future. On the one hand there are extravagant claims that science and technology will provide solutions to all our problems. On the other hand there is fear of science and technology as a juggernaut that could destroy us. Science is more often than not perceived as value free, that is to say as objective and uninfluenced by the values and goals of society and that the task of science and technology is to provide facts. What is done with these facts is a matter for politicians.

But science is not neutral. It is laden with values, some sciences more obviously so than others. Moreover, the very knowledge of science is often a matter of subjective judgment. The great theories of science are not monoliths of truth. They are a combination of facts and hypotheses and subjective judgments subject to further development as ideas and techniques develop. The public has little awareness of these matters. So it attributes to science a degree of objectivity that thinking scientists themselves deny. This leads to inappropriate expectations. Science also is, and is perceived to be, male-dominated. If we are to change the impact of science and technology on the general public we must first know how the general public gets its ideas of science and technology. The main influences are: everyday activities in which we use the products of science and technology, the media, education and the government. All these influences support the dominant view.

Misunderstandings of science by the public extend into the way in which the relations of science and religion are perceived. They are usually seen as separate compartments of knowledge which have little to do with each other except when they clash over rival views such as creationism and evolution. But knowledge is one. Knowledge cannot be divided this way into separate compartments without making great distortions.

The direct beneficial impacts of science on society are obvious. But there are direct impacts which are negative such as the influence of technologies on unemployment and the extent to which resources devoted to science and technology are used for research and development in military activities. These are deeply disturbing influences of science and technology in our society.

The transformation of science for the future

We see a need for a transformation of science itself as well as the need for a better understanding of science by the public. This involves:

1. A deeper appreciation by both scientists and the public of science as value-involved. Some of the values of a "new science" suggested by Everett Mendelsohn are:

— *Modesty*: A moderation of aims and a recognition that choices should replace the arrogance of much contemporary science.

— *Accessibility*: The demystification of scientific knowledge so that it is more accessible to the public, enabling them to participate in important decisions.

— *Non-manipulation*: A non-violent approach to nature which seeks not to manipulate unless absolutely necessary.

— *Harmony with nature*: A concern over the long-term effects of ecological insensitivity, so that one asks if activities will add to or detract from the quality of human and non-human life.

— *Non-sexist*: Equal involvement of women and men.

2. A more unified understanding in which knowledge is not seen as the piling up of one brick upon another but as an indivisible unity. One might have hoped that the churches would have provided a lead in this direction. But with a few exceptions, such as within parts of Eastern Orthodoxy and in some theologies such as process theology, they have not led the way. Instead we find the craving for this sort of understanding is leading people, not to the churches, but to all manner of other groups, some more credible than others. Some, for example, are attracted to Goethe's phenomenology, others to Eastern philosophies; there is the movement that combines mysticism science and philosophy promoted by Ken Wilber and his journal *Revision,* and there is a small group of young Dutch scientists who are exploring the alchemical tradition.

For many scientists the scientific search for order in the universe does not lead to any overall sense of meaning. Nevertheless there is a craving to make some sense of things as a whole and to find a meaning which is both highly personal and at the same time all-embracing. Scientists and teachers should be challenged to look beyond the strictly "scientistic" outlook to a more encompassing search of meaning. Harvard professor Stephen Weinberg in his book *The First Three Minutes* concludes: "The more the universe seems comprehensible, the more it also seems pointless." Is that all there is to be said? A Dutch student recently wrote: "Reading these words for the first time I found them cheerless, indeed tragic." In seeking a deeper meaning the churches could play a decisive role but as yet they are doing very little.

3. A greater emphasis on small-scale technology, a more human technology and stewardship of the resources of the earth and its life-support systems.

4. The application of a transformed science is dependent upon a society which is also in process of transformation towards a more just, participatory and sustainable society. Both processes are inseparable. The sort of economics and politics practised in a society determines very largely the sort of science and technology preached. Many schools of economic thought rely on assumptions ("economic rationality", "the market", etc.) which deliberately exclude moral considerations. Most disturbing is the growing tendency for governments to invoke economic "laws" and the autonomy of the economy to justify highly value-laden policies for industrial and social development. Economic policies that result in harmful pollution of air, food and water, and transport systems

that waste valuable energy are themselves part of the sin of society. Churches should become more aware of the extent to which science and technology have become slaves of economic forces.

5. The churches have a responsibility to seek ways of communicating a new understanding of science and technology to scientists and technologists themselves.

Participation of the public in decision-making and for becoming responsible in science and technology

Participation of the public involves the professions, the labour movement, pressure groups, church groups, political parties and minority groups. This should start in schools and universities in science courses. Students can be given problems involving ethical decisions on topics such as pollution, energy generation, consumption and the like.

In most countries there are institutions which exist to promote communication between scientists, technologists and the general public and which recognize the ethical shortcomings of the dominant view of science. Some of them attempt to involve the public in applied science and technological decision-making. We give some examples here in the hope that they may be applied or adapted to new situations:

1. *Adult education*: The Centro Culturale Jacopo Lombardini is a private school in Italy in which students do not pay fees. The curriculum is more topical and more closely linked to social and technological problems than is usual but the students prepare for state exams. The students' everyday experience of pollution, energy problems, etc. is central to the learning process. There is a two-way flow of information and ideas between teacher and student.

2. *University and society courses* in the Free University of Amsterdam are given by scientific staff of the university in a number of centres in the Netherlands to interested persons and public groups on subjects such as microchips and society, the migrant worker in society, and disarmament. The aim is to provide up-to-date information on matters of general interest to the public and to bring the scientist and the public together.

3. *The project "transformation of science"* undertaken by students and young scientists in Amsterdam. The project is supported by the student pastorate. Its aim is to integrate science within a broader context of understanding that includes meaning as well as order.

4. *Church-sponsored research and study projects*: The society, religion and technology project of the Church of Scotland was set up in 1970 to promote the understanding of problems of science, technology and society, paying special attention to ethical aspects. In the Netherlands the Multidisciplinary Centre for Church and Society has the support of the National Council of Churches. Its three staff members work on issues of social responsibility in science and technology through study groups, conferences and publications. The Protestant churches in the Federal Republic of Germany sponsor the

Forschungsstätte der Evangelischen Studiengemeinschaft (FEST) in Heidelberg. Scientists, philosophers and theologians work together on ethical research and its applications in topics such as genetic counselling and energy policy. Thus the work of such units varies according to whether the stress is on policy or basic research in theology and ethics.

5. *The World Council of Churches' "Hearing on Nuclear Weapons and Disarmament"* is another example of a church body bringing together experts from many disciplines in an open hearing. An open hearing on nuclear energy has recently been organized by the Dutch government.

6. *Science shops*: The "science shop" is a means of bringing scientists, science students and the public together in the Netherlands. They provide a consultancy service in the universities on issues that concern members of the public in science and law. The aim of the science shop is firstly to provide an opportunity for members of the public to call upon the expertise of scientists without cost, and secondly to foster social responsibility among scientists and science students in the university. In this way both the teaching and research activities of the university become related to the needs of society. The science shops are mostly run by students under the supervision of scientists and are supported by the universities. Students can also gain formal credit for their work in the science shop.

7. *The Foundation for Life Sciences and Society in the Netherlands*: This brings to all levels of society insights into present and future research in biology and biological issues (e.g. abortion) that are of importance for society. It provides a service of information and publications to teachers, journalists and any others who wish to be members. These in turn communicate their understanding to a wider public. There are a number of similar centres in other countries.

8. *There are ad hoc meetings of scientists and the public* such as the discussion initiated by the mayor of Cambridge (Mass.) to bring the public into the debate on whether or not to grant permission to build containment facilities for genetic engineering in Harvard University and at MIT.

Participation always involves making scientific and technical information accessible and providing opportunities for its public discussion.

Recommendations

1. In view of the false image of science which is widespread amongst the public we urge the WCC and its member churches and the associations of science teachers to give high priority to fostering a new view of science both among scientists and the general public. It will be a science which is value involved and which will make possible greater conversation with religions and other movements that seek meaning in the universe and that seek to explore the ethical issues arising from scientific developments. The churches must bring their theology into line with a more unified understanding of science, humanity and God.

2. In order to work out the implications of a new science for specific sciences such as biology and physics we urge the churches and universities to give high priority to the development of interdisciplinary centres. The aim of such centres is to see that knowledge may be understood as a unity instead of in terms of separated disciplines. Some centres already exist, such as the Centre for Multi-Disciplinary Studies of Science, Society and Ethics in the Free University of Amsterdam. More are needed and the churches can provide initiatives in establishing them.

3. In view of the high proportion of scientists and technologists who are employed in research and development for military purposes we urge churches to stimulate critical reflection on the ethical implications of military work with those of their members who are involved in it.

4. We urge journalists in the religious media (WCC and member churches) to recognize the growing movement of "science, technology and society" and to reflect this in their journalism.

5. We recommend to the WCC that it makes a major study of the teaching of science in schools and universities in relation to the following question: How can faith meet science so as to relate God to the world in a way which provides meaning and purpose, not just to human life but to the whole universe and all that is in it? We recommend to universities and teachers' colleges that they re-examine the effects of their teaching of science in so far as it leads to a materialistic and mechanistic view of the world, and that they consider contemporary ways in which alternative views which provide room for values and purposes can be introduced into the class room.

SCIENCE EDUCATION IN UNIVERSITIES

SUMMARY OF THE DISCUSSION
HENK VERHOOG

The group on university teaching discussed the relation between science and values, ethics and models of science teaching and the need for an ongoing dialogue between scientists, ethicists and theologians. Special attention was given to the impact of scientific and technological developments on the third world and to the possible role of religious faith. The main theme of this group was the role of ethics in science teaching at the university level.

Edge distinguishes between three models of teaching science, involving three different conceptions of "science":

1. Science as an unproblematic body of knowledge about the natural world; science as theory, transmitted to students within a hierarchical teacher-student relationship.
2. Science as a particular process of enquiry. The emphasis is upon doing creative research. Students may get involved in research itself; there is partnership between teacher and student.
3. Science as a social activity: the acquisition of knowledge for the sake of collective liberation and personal development. Socio-ethical goals are explicitly incorporated in the conception of science itself. Teacher and student collaborate.

It was agreed that the first model dominates in science teaching nowadays and that ethics can only be integrated and made explicit within the third model. Only within the third conception of science does it become clear that ethics is implicit in scientific activity, is part of science itself and not something outside the domain of science. Empiricists and positivists, emphasizing the value-freedom of science, are implicitly accepting a dualistic view of the relation between science and ethics. The result of models 1 and 2 is that students go into the world with very naive expectations, unprepared to tackle the value-issues with which they necessarily come into contact in almost all occupations;

unable to integrate their religious values with their work as scientists. Edge mentioned public controversies such as the recombinant DNA debate in which scientists get involved as advisers. Aikenhead analyzed collective decision-making processes about several social issues involving science and technology. When scientists are challenged they often don't know how to respond. In his paper Aikenhead gave a guiding list of ten items which could be used to detect the technical and the value-element in socio-ethical decision-making. It is a good example of ethical reasoning within the boundaries of science as conceived in model 3. Another example was given by Schroten about euthanasia. He stressed that medical technology has to show its humility and respect towards life. Here we see again that the physician applying technology cannot escape a confrontation with values such as respect for life.

We arrive at the situation that in a science-based society in almost all occupations of scientists they are confronted with a model 3 conception of science whereas they are educated within models 1 and 2. I said almost all occupations. At first sight the university itself seems to be an exception. In many universities since the end of the nineteenth century the emphasis has been on "pure science" (as opposed to applied), value-free research for its own sake. This being the case it is not surprising that this particular conception of science for its own sake is also implemented in the universities' educational systems. It has even led to the distinction between the scientist as scientist and the scientist as citizen. Verhoog emphasized that value-freedom or neutrality is a methodological *a priori* of science (model 2), and this principle of value-freedom should not be confused with or identified with the view that science as a human social activity ought not to take into account the socio-ethical aspects of this activity.

Socio-political neutrality demands of the scientist that he pursue science for its own sake, rather than pursuing it for the solution of social problems. A moral choice is involved here. The choice for methodologically value-free science is itself an ethical choice. This normative premise of university-science is usually not openly stated. If it is openly stated it is usually called the cultural value of science. It becomes evident from the three models identified that the humanistic, cultural value of science is not achieved by merely practising natural science as it is done today in specialized disciplines. The humanistic value appears within the wider cultural context in which science (models 1 and 2) is practised. In this wider cultural context it is a very legitimate question to compare the scientific method with other methods, or to ask for the relation between science and religion.

Considering the relations between science and religion in the context of model 3 it becomes clear that there need not be a conflict or dualism between science and religion. As we have formulated it religious faith may influence the selection of topics, it can lead the science teacher to convey to students a sense of the limitations of science, etc. This may become visible in the science policy of religious-based universities. In state universities the cultural context of fundamental science has changed rapidly during the last few years. The value of science for its own sake is gradually changing into the direction of goal-directed fundamental science. The goals are to an ever greater extent formulated by politicians or industry. So we see that even at universities the climate is changing although it is not self-evident that this change will lead to an integration of the social and ethical aspects in science-teaching. This will only be the case when the "reflexive" attitude, characteristic of model 3, is implemented within science curricula.

When we compare the three models we notice that the conception of science of model 3 includes the other conceptions and not vice versa. The conception of science as a social phenomenon can integrate the educational goals of the other conceptions to a large extent. But once we have opted for conception 1 it becomes almost impossible to integrate conception 3. The choice for 1 automatically leads to dualism between science and ethics, internal and external. This dualistic neo-positivistic approach has permeated the philosophy, sociology and history of science for a very long time, though since Kuhn's *Structure of Scientific Revolutions* the approach has been transcended by many scholars.

In the context of model 3 "contextual values" and "constitutive values" of science (distinctions made in Aikenhead's paper) become integrated. It is not so that the constitutive values are sacrificed for the sake of the contextual values. Science in the sense of model 2 is not becoming "ideological" as is often said. That this is so can best be illustrated by looking at the scheme of the "social cycle" and "empirical cycle" of scientific research (see Manenschijn's paper). To restrict the scientist's responsibility to the empirical cycle (models 1 and 2) means in the case of natural science and technology that the scientist unreflexively puts his scientific results into the hands of the established powers in society. Therefore, one can understand that as soon as scientists or students start questioning model 1 and model 2 this is experienced as a threat to the established institutions in which these larger contextual values are embedded.

This leads us to the question of how the teacher should go ahead if he has opted for model 3 and if there are no institutional barriers. Aikenhead emphasized the intellectual independence of the student as a basic assumption. In ethics this is called the ethical "autonomy" of a person. This means that one can go quite a long way with the process of discovery, of analysis of factual and evaluational elements in science as conceived in model 3. One can compare processes of reasoning in science (model 2) and in ethics as Manenschijn has shown in his paper without leading the student to any particular choice, e.g. that of the teacher himself. Byrne has described an educational unit which can be considered as a model 3 piece of education. The exercise, in which students were divided into three sub-groups representing various interests, was about the use of hot or cool water washing products. The information studied was about energy costs, safety, and pollution. The exercise was not meant to prove one particular socio-ethical point of view but to show students some of the mechanisms and related values that play a role in such discussions. I refer again to Aikenhead's paper, especially the section "Implications for Teaching Science", and the pitfalls which may hinder instruction in this field. We believe that the teaching objective should not be to promote a particular answer but to encourage the recognition of ethical issues, to increase the student's ability in critical thinking and ethical reasoning, and to prepare students for responsible decision-making in an increasingly pluralistic society.

It will take time to get used to thinking and working with model 3 science and education. In the meanwhile we have the situation that most teachers are not really prepared to deal with these issues. This means that a first step towards a change in this situation is to establish a dialogue between scientists, ethicists and others. Good examples are the interdisciplinary workshops mentioned by Ferrer Pí. The aim of these workshops is to help each other in understanding interdisciplinary questions and in discovering new elements in the issues by working together. An important problem in these discussions is the language used within different disciplines. There may be different conceptions of "truth", say scientific and religious, depending upon the language used. Also the difference between scientific and ethical reasoning can be learned in such interdisciplinary workshops. Not only can scientists learn from ethicists but also the other way round. Without knowledge of science and of the actual role of science in society, ethicists may not be able to deal adequately with the issues involved. Another attempt to do something about integrating ethics and professional work is the course on ethics for employees of a commercial bank in Spain (Iuncosa-Carbonell). In this course the emphasis is upon professional responsibility in relation to conscience. The theme of moral responsibility offers a good entrance to the field of ethics because it enables one to discuss the tension between the role responsibility determined by the institution for which one works and a personal sense of responsibility following from the acceptance of ethical norms which may demand that existing institutions be changed to make room for more freedom, justice, and community.

REPORT

Based on the impressive achievements of science and its profound effects on society, the scientific community is by and large still optimistic about the potentialities of science and its capacity to produce a better future. On the other hand there is an indiscriminate pessimism about the impact of science on society among a growing proportion of the population. In this situation we ask in what ways the Christian faith can contribute to a sensitive critique of science and technology that includes a word of hope to a world in crisis. We are concerned about the role of science in building a better world, and the role of ethics in the teaching of science in the university.

Science and values

Science is not a value-free or neutral activity; it is influenced by its cultural, political and economic context, i.e. by contextual values. The directions of scientific research are in part determined by the goals of scientific institutions and of the political and economic institutions which support them. Especially in some sciences (parts of biology, social sciences), the construction of concepts and theories is often influenced by cultural assumptions and ideas, and the determination of objective, value-free facts is more difficult. Furthermore, scientists have a variety of personal motivations which often go unrecognized. What is called the value-neutrality of science is itself a set of methodological or institutional norms (objectivity and universality, freedom of inquiry and open communication), which often conflict with other interests and values.

In their description of the world scientists exclude human values and come up with a simplified universally applicable picture of the world. It is because of the repeatability of its results that science has led to technological achievements. The undeclared and unconscious assumption that science is value-free is a fundamental fallacy in thinking about the relation between science and society. It makes the scientist see only the technical aspects of social problems and neglect the implied moral choices and dilemmas. This holds for both research institutions and universities. It is important for scientists and teachers to be aware of the social and ethical values present in the scientific enterprise and in social decisions about science, and to make explicit the implicit norms and values. Public policies concerning the applications of science can also be judged by such values as justice in the distribution of costs and benefits, and stewardship of the earth and its resources.

Science and technology have brought great intellectual and material benefits to humanity. This has led some people (both within and outside the scientific community) to unlimited confidence in scientific rationality as the source of all understanding, and a reliance on technology as the solution to all human problems. While faith in inevitable progress is less common today when the human and environmental costs of technology are everywhere evident, there is a temptation to neglect the limitations of science by turning it into a new ideology. The science teacher can help students see the need for human wisdom as well as scientific understanding in a world in which science and technology have a dominant position and authority.

Why does the study of science often have a materialistic impact on the outlook of students? Is it the result of preoccupation with science to the exclusion of other areas of experience and interest? Or the result of exclusive reliance on the methods of science? The mechanistic concepts prominent in many sciences since Newton have sometimes been extended into a mechanistic world-view. When random chance and deterministic law were assumed in science, some scientists saw only a universe of law and chance. Such interpretations neglect the selective character of scientific constructs; a limited theory has been extended into a total metaphysical system. In responding to the need for a more holistic understanding we can point to the importance of social, aesthetic and religious experience. We believe that both the churches and the universities have a responsibility to help science students to see the findings of science within a larger framework of meaning; both in their own way have neglected this task.

Ethics and models of science teaching

Consideration was given to three models for the teaching of science:

1. *Science as content and information*: Students are inducted into science by exposure to exemplary problem solutions and techniques. It is assumed that topics are discrete; course work is guided by a segmented syllabus, and there is one "correct answer" to every question. Teacher-student relationships are hierarchical; the intention is to achieve a flow of essentially unproblematic "facts" and information from teacher to student.

2. *Science as a creative process of inquiry*: In the second model science is thought of not as a product but primarily as a process of inquiry. Rather than a "body of knowledge" to be transmitted from student to teacher, it is seen as a potentially generalized mode of inquiry, a process of rational and experimental exploration in which students can participate with the assistance of teachers. Here notions of the pluralistic nature of science and the relativity of truth-claims are accommodated.

3. *Science as socially relevant knowledge*: In the third model the relevance of science to individual development and human needs is stressed. Here science encompasses both results and methods but from the perspective of the way science is used. The science that is learned develops outwards from the student's individual interests and abilities. Science is seen as a product of many contingencies, and not as a body of abstract principles to be transmitted.

We recognize that the choice among these models may vary greatly according to the age and level of the individual, the academic discipline, and the institutional context. We agree that the choice of models also reflects ethical judgments concerning the goals of education and the personal and intellectual consequences of differing patterns of student-teacher relationship. We also agree that some components of the first model—especially its concern for fundamental principles, intellectual rigour and objective analysis—should be included in all science teaching. At the same time it is desirable that all students at some point should consider the social context of science.

We disagree, however, as to the extent to which features of the differing models should be emphasized. For some the first model remains central in the training of scientists, especially at the university level, but it should be supplemented by additional separate courses, and by carefully chosen units within standard courses in science. For others a more radical shift towards the second or third models is called for. It was pointed out that as long as examinations are designed from the perspective of the first model, and structures of reward and authority are dominated by its assumptions, students will perceive contextual questions as peripheral. Cooperation and compromise among adherents of different models will be like cooperation between the lion and the lamb. In the third world in particular there is great interest in teaching science from the perspective of its relevance to human needs.

The choice among models raises far-reaching questions. Pedagogical changes require institutional changes in order to be effective. Even with new curriculum materials, teachers find it difficult to use methods differing from those in which they were trained. There is some debate as to which model will attract the most able students and produce the most socially responsible scientists. Some representation from the second and third models is essential for the recognition that science is value-laden and that scientific theories are social constructions. Moreover, these models encourage the student to place the study of science in a wider framework. These alternative models are also important in understanding the interaction of scientists with the public, especially in the case of policy controversies.

Dialogue between scientists and theologians

In the course of pursuing their work scientists are confronted with ethical dilemmas which have consequences for themselves, their colleagues and experimental subjects, and sometimes for the whole social order. To ensure that these dilemmas are properly understood we believe it is necessary that there be rigorous, ongoing dialogue among scientists, moral philosophers and theologians. The success of such a dialogue will depend on the openness of scientists to such engagement and the willingness of ethicists and theologians to become more acquainted with science, its methodology, its problems, its content and its personal and social implications.

At the same time an important contribution to the education of both future scientists and non-scientists can be made as they are introduced in their study of science to these ethical dilemmas. The teaching objective should not be to promote a particular answer but to encourage the recognition of ethical issues, to increase the student's ability in critical thinking and ethical reasoning, and to prepare students for responsible decision-making in an increasingly pluralistic society. To accomplish this will require that science teachers do some serious study in ethics, or work closely with philosophers or theologians interested in ethical theory and application.

Science, technology and ethics in the third world

Developing countries have become increasingly aware of the need for western science and technology as a means to progress and enhancement of economic and political wellbeing. The mechanistic world-view implicit in science is usually incompatible with the traditional systems of the developing countries where life is perceived as a whole.

In transfer of science and technology to third world countries an awareness of the depersonalizing effect of western science would facilitate assessment of the types of technology that are best suited for implementation. These countries feel left behind in levels of scientific and technological competence, and in their hurry to catch up they are prone to many pitfalls which at present may not seem to be of much consequence to them in their over-riding desire for progress. This makes it necessary that the western assessment of the impact of science and technology should reflect a global concern. Current growth in such fields as micro-electronics and biotechnology are increasing the gap between industrial and developing countries.

The role of religious faith

In the past religious authorities have tried to dictate scientific conclusions. Today many Christians are aware that their legitimate concern for science should not result in a repetition of past mistakes. Religious faith may influence the selection of the topics which the scientist or the public considers most important for research, and it may influence the kind of concept or hypothesis which is being proposed. But the choice among competing scientific theories must be decided by the scientific community itself. However, religious faith can lead the science teacher to convey to students a sense of the limitations of science and humility concerning the tentative and selective character of its concepts and theories.

The Christian tradition has held distinctive views about human fulfilment and human nature which are relevant to judgments about applied science and technology and the institutions which control them. Specific social decisions and policies involving technology can be analyzed in relation to such values of justice, participation and sustainability. How are costs, benefits and risks distributed? Who has a voice in the decision? How will the environment and future generations be affected?

Recommendations

— *To universities in general* :

We urge that formal instruction and practical experience in moral reasoning and ethical decision-making be included in science curricula, at both the undergraduate and graduate levels.

— *To universities and professional scientific associations*:

We call upon the academic and professional scientific communities to defend the rights of teachers and professional scientists who, in the pursuit of ethical responsibility in their teaching and research activities, challenge traditional pedagogical and research practices.

— *To universities involved in international development education and research, and to government departments of international development*:

In the light of the great danger of naïve and potentially destructive transfer of technology, we strongly recommend that every effort be taken—

especially in close collaboration with third world peoples—to ensure that the planning for and evaluation of development education and technology transfer be carried out in such a way as to advance the values and quality of life in the third world and contribute to peace and justice.

—To UNESCO and to the International Association of Universities:

We recommend that, in order to stress the great importance of teaching ethics within science curricula, a special institute or department be created within these organizations to promote and advance such activity.

— To theological faculties in universities and graduate centres of religion:

We urge that attention be given in the curricula to ethical issues arising from science and technology, and to the relation between faith and science.

— To the World Council of Churches and its member churches:

We urge that the churches and the WCC encourage an awareness of the ethical and social problems which confront the world in this age of science and high technology, and give greater attention in their witness to the ways in which science-based technology may be used to enhance the quality of life for all people and contribute to global justice, participation and sustainability.

We urge that continued discussion of the relation between faith and science and analysis of theological and ethical issues raised by science and technology should be high among WCC programme priorities in the future. We recommend that the concern of this workshop for the role of ethics in science education in western Europe be continued via similar workshops in other regions.

SCIENCE EDUCATION IN SECONDARY SCHOOLS AND TEACHER TRAINING INSTITUTES: INTEGRATED REPORT

Issues of science and ethics, when seen from the point of view of the education of children, raise questions concerning the role and responsibilities of the science teacher not only in terms of the transmission of science, but also in relation to the general goals of education in our societies. That is, the justification for the inclusion of science in the curriculum, and the way it is treated, is derived not only from science, but also from the needs of children, future adults and society. The aims of science education should arise from within this context.

A consideration of the aims of science education within schools is pertinent to teacher trainers as well as to school teachers since the aims of science teacher training are directly related to work in schools. That is not to say that teacher training institutions must simply reflect the needs of schools; they may be able to take an innovatory role—but this will only be effective if it is related in some way to work in classrooms. Teacher training is concerned not only with the preparation of new teachers, but also, through in-service work, with serving teachers. Both teacher trainers and science teachers are interested, in the final analysis, in the same thing, that is the work that goes on in science classrooms.

The particular responsibility of science teachers involves developing methodologies which make accessible to children that area of human experience called science so that the children can come to understand this knowledge in its cultural context, and develop further their interest if they wish. The ethical dimension of science and the possible needs of future adults add to the responsibility of science teachers to extend their teaching methods to enable the study of issues of science and society to arise in their science programmes. This means that it is important that we should not consider science education in isolation, but in relation to moral education in particular.

The perceived need for an ethical dimension to school science is reflective of the social impact of technical change and also of changing ideas about the nature of science.

Three elements of technical and social change are seen to be of significance in relation to science education:

1. Development of new technologies relating for example to consumer products, transport, communication, information storage and retrieval, health, food, and defence. Such technologies are likely to have worldwide and longstanding influences.
2. Many societies are becoming more pluralistic, individuals and groups having different perceptions of individual and societal wellbeing, different definitions of benefits and costs, and different images of the future. The differences augment and magnify social conflicts.
3. In many countries more citizens are involved in public decision-making. In many issues where such decisions need to be made, scientific and technological judgments are involved as well as political, moral, economic and legal ones.

Contemporary science education at the secondary level is often based on the idea that science is neutral, value-free and isolated from questions of values and ethics. There is an emphasis on the teaching of a specific body of knowledge and skills related to the needs of future scientists working in a value-free situation. Little attention is paid to the needs of future citizens.

The dominant values of most science education at present are of a constitutive character; they are inherent to the internal system of the discipline. Contextual values which affect scientific and technological enterprises such as those which influence fields of research to be funded, those which are involved in policy discussions on a technological implementation and value influences on research methodologies (e.g. experimenting with minds or human subjects) are not usually included. This is reflected in the textbooks and also, importantly, in public examinations which significantly influence work in science classrooms.

Scientific "objectivity" is one of the constitutive values communicated to students in science textbooks. However, science textbooks themselves have been shown to camouflage subtle value-laden messages. For example it is often implied that social problems can be solved simply with more scientific knowledge and innovative technology.

The experience of science, in the case of most secondary science teachers, is likely to have been a positivist one. Inevitably this will colour a science teacher's views about science education, and may help explain why many science teachers find it difficult to deal with subjective issues and moral reasoning in their classroom work.

It was agreed that there must be a change in emphasis in science education from simply teaching scientific knowledge and skills to learning how to use knowledge and skills in personal and social life, and that this should take into account contemporary views about the nature of scientific knowledge. Such a change of emphasis suggests the need to consider the role of schools in relation to moral education.

Secondary schools have a responsibility for moral education. The aims of moral education are to enable pupils to achieve the following:

1. to form, articulate and express their own value judgments;
2. to distinguish between different points of view (law, morality, self-interest, religion);
3. to take their own decisions, justifying those referring to norms, values and principles;
4. to learn the difference between the moral norms, values and principles one personally subscribes to (personal morality), and the moral norms, values, and principles to which one is expected to agree as a member of a group or society (public morality);
5. to learn the difference between personal decisions in the private sphere and collective decisions in the public sphere;
6. to accept the existence of different moral opinions and systems of morality;
7. to accept the right of other persons to hold opinions different from one's own.

The following skills, competences and attitudes, are necessary in order to realize those aims:

1. analytical skills as tools for a more articulate and consistent way of justifying moral judgments and of describing the process of moral reasoning;
2. communicative skills: listening to others; the ability to paraphrase another's point of view and the capacity to connect with another person's opinion;
3. imagination and empathy.

The task of moral education cannot be assigned to one area. Ethical questions arise in most areas, e.g. history, science, religion, literature. Moral education can only be fruitful when it is related to concrete and practical questions.

Teaching in all disciplines can contribute to moral education, but the contribution to be expected may be different from discipline to discipline. Moral education is relevant to science education because many contemporary social and political problems are related to science and technology. Science education is relevant to moral education because in moral reasoning not only norms, values and principles play a role, but also factual judgments. Science is an important source of factual information that pupils should be able to weigh critically.

At the secondary school level the introduction of ethical aspects in science education depends strongly on the teachers. A distinction can be made between the following groups of teachers:

1. those who are against introducing ethical aspects in science education;
2. those who think it is not possible;
3. those who are willing but don't know how to do it;
4. those who try but meet a lot of problems;
5. those who are successful.

We are not dealing here with group 5; others may be able to learn from them if written or audiovisual description of their work is made available. Our concern is the reasons behind teachers' attitudes in groups 1 to 4. We identified several factors which play a negative role:

1. overloaded science curricula pressurized by an oppressive examination system;
2. a pedagogical climate in the schools which is not favourable to moral development;
3. lack of training in moral reasoning among science teachers;
4. inability of teachers to deal with student activities which promote moral development so that students have little opportunity to face the consequences of their moral choices, and so are rarely challenged;
5. resistance by teachers to changes in their role in classroom; fear of losing respect by shifting responsibilities to students when using new teaching methods;
6. lack of communication and cooperation between teachers in different disciplines;
7. lack of understanding among teachers of the contemporary nature of science and technology;
8. inability of teachers to assess progress in moral reasoning.

What are we actually asking of science teachers when we suggest they extend their methodologies?

We may expect science teachers to be competent in their own field of knowledge and in practical and technical skills related to their field, and to have sufficient understanding of the theory and practice of general education, e.g. the psychological, sociological and moral context of learning and development. Science teaching has traditionally been seen to be largely unproblematic and relatively objective. A broader view of science and its role in education has changed this situation, especially of what we expect of science teachers.

We believe that secondary school teachers should acquire the following competences:

1. the capability to communicate the possibilities and the limitations of one's own field of study;
2. the ability to relate one's discipline to other school disciplines;
3. the capability to place one's own discipline within the context of the child's world;
4. willingness to deal with the more public aspects of one's material e.g. as reflected in newspapers;
5. skills in handling issue studies in the field of science and society.

In practice it is not reasonable to expect every science teacher to deal with all the social and ethical issues related to his or her field of study!

Implications for science education

1. In secondary science education we must:
a. adopt as a primary educational objective the training of pupils for active participation in decision-making processes in a democratic society;
b. hence avoid a too early and too rigid division of the complete group of children of this age into two separate groups of (1) pre-scientists, and (2) pupils without professional aspirations towards science and technology;
c. realize this by (1) postponing the moment of "streaming" as long as possible, and (2) presenting—even after the establishment of separate streams—some part of science education to mixed groups of children;
d. recognize that students should not be forced to have an opinion; this is a personal matter and should be respected.

2. With respect to the subject matter of secondary science education and the organization of the content of curricula, the following are recommended:
a. concentration on the scientific and technological environment of the pupils;
b. thematic organization of syllabi;
c. focus on the problems of "science, technology and society";
d. development of a fuller image of scientific knowledge and of the role of science and technology in society;
e. integration of the discussion of ethical issues and science education at relevant points of the curriculum.

Implications for teacher education

In considering teacher education in respect to science and ethics there are two inter-related aspects:
1. the development of science teachers' awareness of the nature of science and its social, political, economic and moral context;
2. the provision of opportunities to develop skills for creating methods of teaching which take into account the ethical dimensions of science.

Recommendations

1. That there should be a change of emphasis in science education in schools to encourage more learning about how to use knowledge and skills in personal and social life, and that this should be reflected in public examinations.
2. That pre-service and in-service training for teachers be provided to equip (a) science teachers with the necessary skills for developing methods of teaching which take into account the ethical dimensions of science and (b) all teachers with a sufficient understanding of science to enable them to work cooperatively with teachers in category (a).

LIST OF PARTICIPANTS

van AALST, Dr H.F. (Netherlands) — Highschool Project Advising Group (A.P.V.O.II)

AIKENHEAD, Dr Glen S. (Canada) — Department of Curriculum Studies, University of Saskatchewan, Saskatoon

BARBOUR, Prof. Ian G. (USA) — Department of Religion, Carleton College, Northfield, Minn.

BIJKER, Dr W.E. (Netherlands) — "De Boerderij", Technical University, Twente, Enschede

BIRCH, Prof. Charles (Australia) — Department of Biology University of Sydney

BIRFELDER, Dr E.J. (Netherlands) — Institute for Bio-Sciences and Society Leiden

BOCKEMÜHL, Dr Jochen (FRG) — Forschungslaboratorium am Goetheanumm, Dornach Switzerland

BOEKER, Dr Egbert (Netherlands) — Department of Physics, Faculty of Science, Free University, Amsterdam

BYRNE, Dr M. (UK) — Polytechnic, Newcastle-upon-Tyne

van der CINGEL, Prof. N.A. (Netherlands) — Department of Didactics of Biology University of Groningen

COMBA, Mr Giovanni (Italy) — Centro Culturale Jacopo Lombardini Milan

DAVIS, Dr Howard H. (UK) — Church of Scotland Society, Religion and Technology Project, Edinburgh

DALDJOENI, Prof. Nathanael (Indonesia) — Department of Social Geography Christian University, Satya Wacana, Salatiga, Java

DUPRE, Dr Franco (Italy)	Department of Physics, University "La Sapienza", Rome
EDGE, Prof. David O. (UK)	Science Studies Unit, University of Edinburgh
van ERKELENS, Dr H. (Netherlands)	Institute of Theoretical Physics University of Amsterdam
EIJKELHOF, Dr Harrie (Netherlands)	Project Curriculum Development Physics (PLON), Laboratory Vaste Stof, Utrecht
FERRER PI, Prof. P., SJ (Spain)	Centro Loyola de Estudios y Communicación Social, Madrid
GOSLING, Dr David (UK)	Department of Theology University of Hull
GRAVENBERCH, Dr F.L. (Netherlands)	National Institute for Curriculum Development
HILHORST, Rev. M.T. (Netherlands)	Student Pastor, Technical University Delft
HOEBEL-MÄVERS, Dr M. (FRG)	Department of Education University of Hamburg
HORTAL, Prof. A. (Spain)	Department of Ethics University of Madrid
HÜBNER, Prof. Jürgen (FRG)	Forschungsstätte der Evangelischen Studiengemeinschaft (FEST) Heidelberg
van HUIS, Dr C. (Netherlands)	Department of Chemistry, Institute for Teachers Education VL-VU Amsterdam
İUNCOSA CARBONELL, Prof. A (Spain)	Department of Ethics and Sociology, Faculty of Philosophy University of Barcelona
KEIDING, Ms Ingelise (Denmark)	Dental College, Copenhagen
KIRSCHENMANN, Dr P.P. (FRG)	Philosophy of the Natural Sciences Free University, Amsterdam
de LANGE, Rev. S. (Netherlands)	Students Chaplain Free University, Amsterdam
LICHT, Dr Pieter (Netherlands)	Department of Physics, Faculty of Science, Free University Amsterdam
LINDBERG, Dr E. (Sweden)	Free Church Educational Institute

MANENSCHIJN, Prof. Gerrit (Netherlands) — Department of Ethics
Faculty of Theology
Free University, Amsterdam

PARSONAGE, Dr Robert R. (USA) — Education in the Society, National Council of Churches, USA

PLEHN, Dr Franz (FRG) — Lecturer in Mathematics and Physics, Berlin

PORTELE, Prof. Gerhard (FRG) — Interdisciplinary Centre for High School Didactics, University of Hamburg

PRITCHARD, Dr A.J. (UK) — Department of Education University of Southampton

PRONK, Dr P. (Netherlands) — Department of Biology
Institute for Teachers Education
VL-VU Amsterdam

RANTA, Dr Osmo (Finland) — Education Counsellor
Department of Sciences and Universities, Ministry of Education

van ROODEN, Dr C.D. (Netherlands) — Science Information Officer Free University, Amsterdam

ROT, Mr G. (Netherlands) — Free University, Amsterdam

SCHERMER, Prof. Alfred K.F. (Netherlands) — Department of Biological Education
Faculty of Biology
Free University, Amsterdam

SCHROTEN, Dr E. (Netherlands) — Department of Theology University of Utrecht

SCHULZE, Dr B. (FRG) — Evangelical Student Parish
Head Office, German Student Christian Movement

SIMMERS, Dr I. (Netherlands) — Department of Geology, Faculty of Science, Free University, Amsterdam

SINGH, Dr Narendra (India) — C.F.T.R.I., Mysore

SLAGTER, Dr K. (Netherlands) — Department of Mathematics and Science, Protestant Institute for Teachers Education, Zwolle

STAFLEU, Dr M.D. (Netherlands) — Department of Physics, Institute for Teachers Education, Utrecht

STRAUGHAN, Prof. R.R. (UK) — Philosophy of Education University of Reading

THAIRU, Dr Henry M. (Kenya)	Department of Chemistry, Kenyatta University College, Nairobi
TUININGA, Dr Eric J. (Netherlands)	Institute for Applied Scientific Research, Free University, Amsterdam
van der VALK, Dr A.E. (Netherlands)	Project Curriculum Development Physics
VERHOOG, Dr Henk (Netherlands)	Institute for Theoretical Biology University of Leiden

Staff

ABRECHT, Dr Paul	Church and Society, World Council of Churches (until 31 December 1983)
BORN, Dr Piet	Department of Physics, Faculty of Science, Free University, Amsterdam
MUSSCHENGA, Dr A.W.	Interdisciplinary Centre for the Study of Science, Society and Religion Free University, Amsterdam
STALSCHUS, Christa	Church and Society World Council of Churches
THOLEN, Leonore	Interdisciplinary Centre for the Study of Science, Society and Religion Free University, Amsterdam
van der VELDEN, Drs H.	Office of the Vice-Chancellor Free University, Amsterdam